The Beginner's Guide to
Fitness

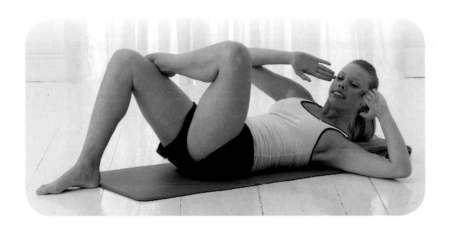

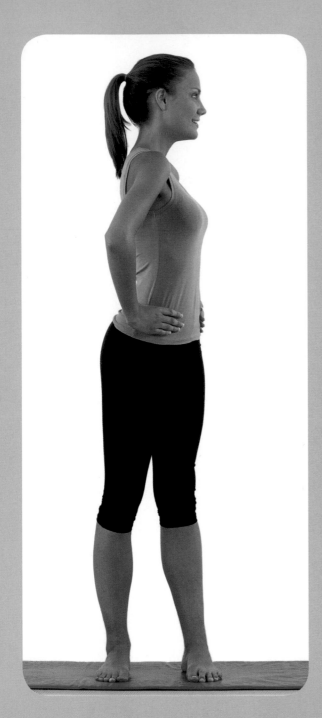

First published by Parragon in 2011

Parragon
Chartist House
15-17 Trim Street
Bath BA1 1HA, UK

www.parragon.com

Designed by Design Principals, Warminster

ISBN 978-1-4454-5641-6

Printed in China

Photography credits: Ian Parsons, all exercise pictures; iStockphoto 10, 12, 13, 14, 15, 24, 27, 28, 30, 31, 32, 33, 105, 140

Caution
Please check with your doctor/therapist before attempting these workouts, particularly if you have an injury, are pregnant, or have just had a baby. It is recommended that new mothers wait at least six weeks postpartum before participating in exercise (12 weeks if it was a Caesarean birth). If you feel any pain or discomfort at any point, please stop exercising immediately and seek medical advice.

The Beginner's Guide to
Fitness

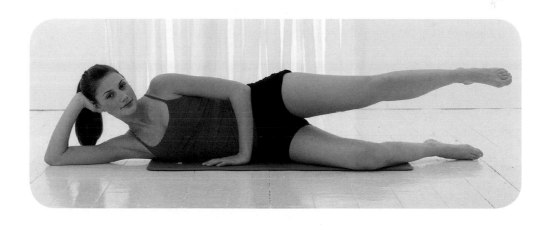

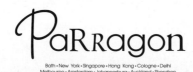

Bath · New York · Singapore · Hong Kong · Cologne · Delhi
Melbourne · Amsterdam · Johannesburg · Auckland · Shenzhen

contents

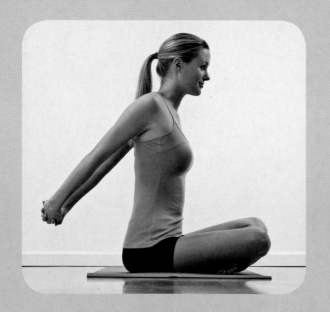

1 starting out

2 chest & back

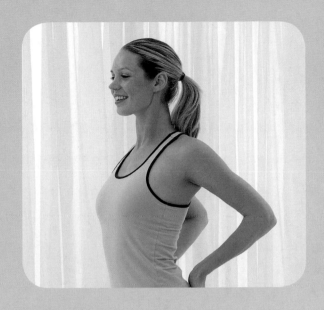

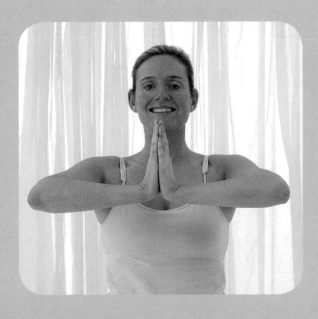

3 arms & shoulders

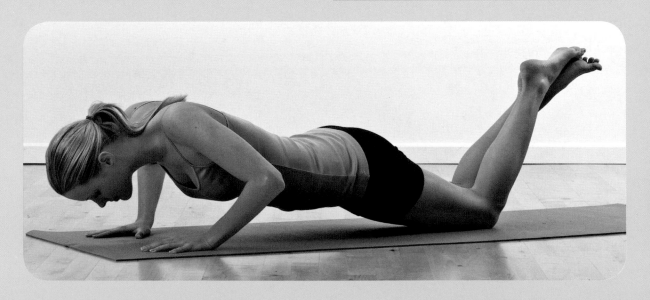

4 stomach

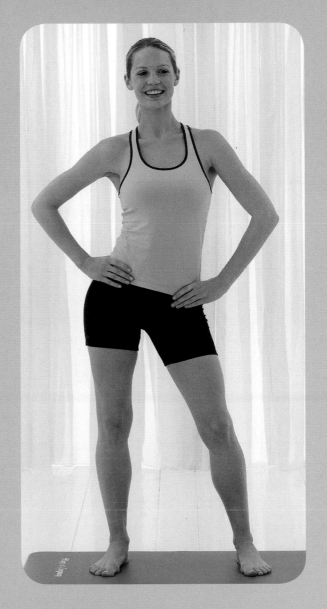

5 legs & buttocks

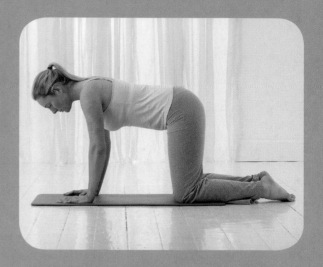

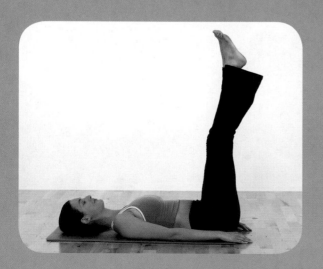

6 core stability

7 exercise planner

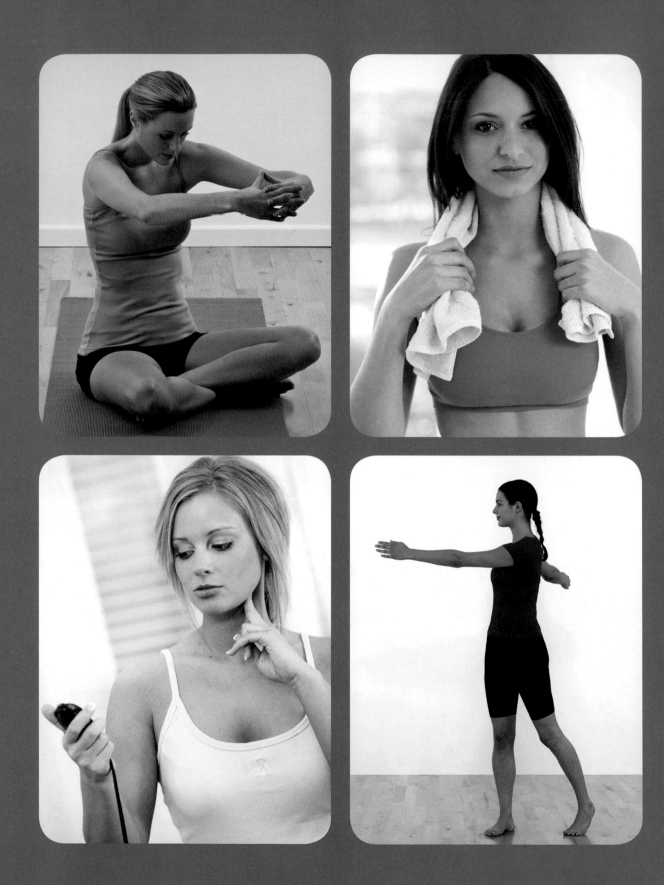

1

starting out

The following pages will help you understand how your body works, and explain how you can improve your health and fitness. There's information on what you need to do before you start, including safety tips, fitness options and creating the right environment, so you can exercise safely. Plus, you'll find out how to improve your posture, a crucial part in any fitness plan.

introduction

If you want to start on the road to getting fit without spending hours in the gym, this is the book for you. The old saying "no pain, no gain" is often true, but the exercises aren't meant to be a daily chore, instead, you should enjoy each day and look forward to trying new experiences.

The best way to get and keep fit is to have a daily routine of regular exercises that combine all the muscle groups. This will bring you noticeable benefits, help you achieve a healthier life, and make you feel good as well.

While this fitness routine will bring you and your body many benefits, those benefits can be greatly increased if you are aware that what goes into your body and how you treat it also affects your fitness. Also, a fit body needs a fit mind, because when you are doing daily exercises you will require determination and motivation.

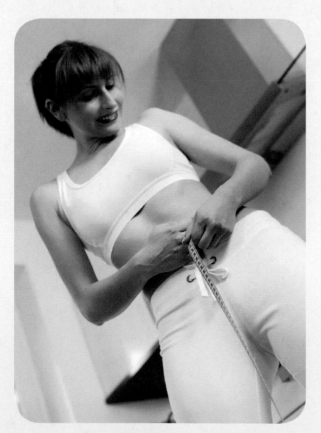

This book covers a wide range of information that explains how to achieve a healthy lifestyle, and contains all the exercises (with instructions and a 12-week plan) that you will need to make a real difference to your overall fitness levels and general well-being.

As well as targeting all the body zones, the stretching and core stability exercises offer a practical range of beneficial routines. So, even if your fitness goals change, this book will still be useful. You don't need any expensive equipment for the majority of the exercises, and can choose to buy an exercise ball for the core stability routines if you want.

All the exercises have been tried and tested by experts in the field and have been found to be very effective. They really do work, so let's get started!

Great reasons for getting fitter

Apart from the obvious benefit of improving your overall health and appearance, taking time to exercise and care for your body will really pay dividends in many other ways. Strengthening your muscles will improve your balance and posture, and increase your flexibility, helping to keep your body in tip-top condition as you get older. As an added bonus, you'll find it easier to control your weight, because muscles burn more calories than fat.

Exercise is also known to boost levels of "happy hormones" (endorphins) in the brain, making you feel more cheerful and relaxed, with a higher sense of self-esteem. Endorphins also beat stress, so you'll not only be a joy to work with, but you're also more likely to perform to your best abilities. And, when you're feeling optimistic, you're more likely to make healthy food choices, which will further help you to achieve your goals.

> **As well as toning and strengthening muscles, exercise can:**
> • Improve your overall physical and mental well-being.
> • Help prevent heart disease, strokes, and type 2 diabetes.
> • Reduce high blood cholesterol and high blood pressure.
> • Prevent arthritis from setting in, help improve bad circulation, and guard against osteoporosis.
> • Relieve stress and anxiety-related problems and improve sleep problems.

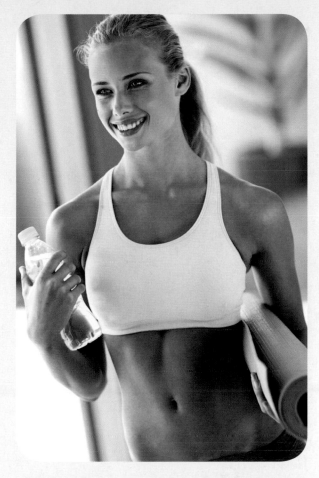

How to exercise

The key to a successful exercise routine is to maintain a regular program. This book combines warm-ups, exercises, and cool-downs into daily routines that are designed to take around 20 minutes, enabling you to fit a workout into even your busiest day. Exercises are grouped into suggested programs at the end of the book, but you can mix and match your own if you want. Building muscle tone doesn't happen overnight, but the beauty of these short routines is that you won't become bored or burned out. Keep it up and you'll discover that finding the time to exercise every day really will make a difference.

We recommend that, before you begin, you thoroughly read the different exercises you want to complete, so you won't waste time wondering exactly how to do them when you start. Remember to spend time warming up, then move straight on to the exercise plan and, once you've finished, on to the cool-down stretches and exercises.

When to exercise

For most people, exercising in the morning is best, when you are refreshed after a night's sleep. Your body is very receptive to exercise in the morning—since it tends to be done on an empty stomach, it forces your body to use its fat reserves. Exercising at this time also jump-starts your metabolism and helps keep you burning calories throughout the day.

However, you may find yourself having to exercise at other times instead of in the morning. For instance, if you have young children, you may well choose to exercise when they are at school or playgroup. The most important thing is to choose a time that is convenient for you and with which you feel comfortable.

Before you start

As with all exercise programs, if you have not exercised for a while, are a complete beginner or had or do have a medical problem, you should discuss this workout plan with your doctor before you start. This is important in order to rule out any health conditions that may prevent you from taking part. Hopefully, you'll be given the green light and a pat on the back, and then there'll be no stopping you!

the way to fitness

No more excuses about starting tomorrow or next week—there's no time like today. Once you have decided to undertake a fitness program, rest assured that you will not regret it, so start planning now and let's work toward your dream of achieving a leaner and fitter body!

The exercises in this book are all relatively easy to follow and perform. If practiced correctly and regularly, they will help you improve your physical and mental well-being and strengthen muscle tone, without it costing a fortune or having to spend hours working out in the gym.

All-round fitness

By following the exercise plans featured later on (see page 210), you will greatly improve your fitness levels, but if you really want to get fit, then you'll need to make sure your diet is healthy too. Also, it would pay dividends to include some activity that raises your heartbeat for at least 15 minutes at a time.

Take the time to read the pages that deal with these points later on. You'll find just a few simple changes to your daily routine can make all the difference.

Starting off

If you're a beginner, you may want to ease yourself gently into the exercise plan and do less repetitions. That's fine if you do, but just remember to be persistent and your efforts will pay off. Soon enough, you'll find that your body will be better able to cope with the routine and, when this happens, you'll know you've made amazing progress. Just stay positive, enthusiastic, and optimistic and you'll reap the rewards.

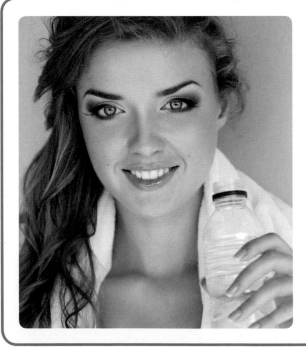

Tips for good practice

Exercising alone means that you don't have a teacher to help you ensure that you practice carefully and so you will need to take full responsibility for your own safety. Make sure you:

- Always do both warm-up and cool-down exercises for at least five minutes to make sure that your heart rate changes slowly and you don't hurt any muscles.
- Never "work through the pain" when exercising; you can only hurt yourself.
- Drink plenty of water during and after your workout to prevent dehydration and muscle stiffness.
- Don't rush the moves—think about what you're doing; it's quality not just quantity.
- Wear appropriate clothing that allows you to move freely and comfortably.
- Follow an exercise program that meets your needs, but make sure that your needs and goals are realistic.

What to wear

Wearing the right gear can make a huge difference to your performance. It's vitally important that you don't just roll out of bed and get started while you're still in your pajamas. Not only might this restrict your movement, but you could trip over baggy clothes, for example, and you won't be in the right frame of mind for exercise.

A breathable Lycra sports top or a fitted T-shirt coupled with stretchy leggings or shorts are the ideal combination. You can pick up some great clothes in a sportswear store but, if you're on a budget, an old pair of tracksuit pants and a fitted tank top should be just fine. The good news is that exercising at home means that you won't be seen by friends or colleagues in less-than-flattering attire.

What you'll need

Equipment: You don't need a great deal of equipment to do the exercises in this book, although there are a few things that may be worth purchasing. You may want to buy a padded exercise mat to work on, because it will help to stop you from slipping on the floor, as well as being a comfortable surface for exercise, and you can also invest in some dumbbells that you feel comfortable using (ask a sales assistant to help you choose a suitable starting weight). If you don't have the cash, a can of beans makes a good dumbbell because it's easy to hold.

For the core stability routines, we recommend using an exercise ball for variation, but you can begin without this if you want.

Make sure you have an alarm clock or wristwatch on hand to help you time the exercises so you know you are doing them for the correct amount of time.

Space: Make sure you clear a space that is big enough for you to move freely in—that means one where you can fully extend your arms and legs without hitting anything. This may involve a bit of furniture reshuffling, but clearing a space especially for exercise and using it every day means you're more likely to stick to the plan as you get used to the routine.

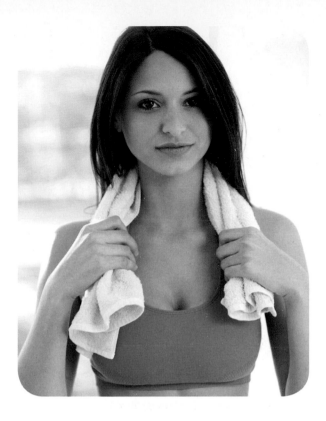

Starting and stopping

Warming up is very important—if you don't warm up, you are likely to injure yourself because your muscles, tendons, and ligaments will be taut. The routines assume that you will have warmed up beforehand—this can be as simple as running on the spot for a few minutes followed by some stretches.

Just as important as warming up before exercising is cooling down afterward. As well as helping to prevent dizziness and a sudden drop in body temperature, cooling down realigns working muscles to their normal position in order to avoid tightness and stiffness.

See pages 18 and 19 for a more in-depth explanation of these crucial stages.

Reps and sets

Muscle-building exercises are done as a series of repetitions (reps). One repetition equals one exercise. A set is a group of repetitions and usually consists of

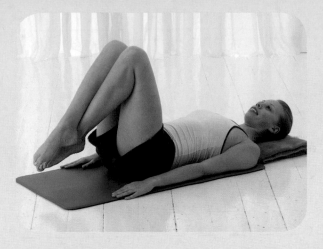

Breathing

The correct way to breathe when exercising is to breathe in slowly through your nose (notice how your abdominal cavity rises as you do so), and breathe out slowly through your mouth. Make sure you continue to breathe in and out regularly throughout. And don't hold your breath—this will cause blood pressure to rise, which can be dangerous.

Keeping elbows and knees soft

If an exercise requires you to extend your arms or legs, remember always to keep elbows and knees "soft" (slightly bent). It will prevent you from getting injured.

eight reps. The aim of repeating exercises is to work until your muscles feel tired, and over time this will strengthen them so that they can work even harder. It's important that you don't stop for more than a minute between exercises. Shorter recovery periods result in better muscles all round and improved muscle endurance. So keep going!

If you do feel any discomfort while carrying out any of the exercises, it's important that you stop what you're doing immediately and take a break. If you ever experience a nagging pain, or feel sick, dizzy, or unusually out of breath at any time while doing the exercises, simply stop and book an appointment with your doctor to rule out any underlying health problems that might be causing the discomfort. It might put your workout plan on hold for a while, but it's best to be safe when it comes to your health.

If your muscles feel sore at any time (if you're not used to exercise, you're most likely to experience this during the first few days of doing the plan), then take some time out to rest until your muscles feel good enough to get going again. As long as you pick up from where you left off and finish the plan without any major disruptions, the effects will be the same.

Lastly, keep a bottle of water close by—keeping hydrated means the muscles work better and you'll be less likely to get a cramp.

Spine in neutral

For some of the exercises, you will be asked to keep your spine in neutral. This means making sure your spine is

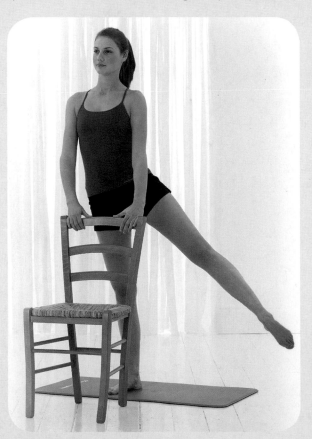

in the right position when you are exercising, which will help you get much better results. The panel at right explains the correct way to achieve this position.

Posture

Having good posture makes all the exercises easier to do and more effective too. On pages 22 to 25 we detail how you can improve your standing and sitting postures, but here are a few specific points to remember while exercising.

Good posture results from your spine maintaining its natural curve, without sagging. If your posture is incorrect, every movement you make will be inefficient, leading to weakness, aching joints and muscles, and an increased risk of injury.

Test your posture by standing on one leg—you should be able to balance without wobbling. Even if you do wobble, the good news is that certain exercises in this book, such as those in the stomach and chest and back sections, will naturally improve your posture because they strengthen the major muscles (the core muscles) that support your body.

The basic thing to remember is, if you're standing, imagine your spine is extended beyond your head up toward the sky and that someone is pulling on the end to make you stand to attention, a little like a puppet on a string. Make sure your shoulders are relaxed—an easy way to check is to roll them backward a few times. This will help you find their natural resting place.

Another point to watch out for is that your stomach muscles are "engaged" at all times, which basically means that they are pulled in, nice and tight. This will automatically prevent your back from curving, making the exercises more effective and guarding you against injury. Make sure you keep all this in mind at all times when exercising.

Sensible targets

Once you have decided to work toward a better level of fitness, you will not regret it. Just don't become too

> ## The neutral position
>
> ### Standing in Neutral Spine
> Stand with your feet hip distance apart and turn your toes slightly outward. Make sure that your body weight is evenly distributed between the feet as well as between the front and back regions of the foot. Roll the foot inward and outward to find the point where the weight of the body is centered. Keep the head straight and level. Try to keep the spine straight but do not over arch the back. The shoulders should be straight and level to the floor.
>
> ### Lying on Your Back in Neutral Spine
> Lie on your back with your knees bent and feet on the floor, hip distance apart. The ankles, knees, and hips should be aligned. The knees should be stable and the lower back touching the floor should feel the weight of the body. The shoulders and back of your ribs should be touching the floor and you should feel the weight of your upper body on them. The center of the back should naturally lift off the floor. The neck should be lengthened away from the body.
>
> ### The following points should be kept in mind during Neutral Position:
> • The ankles, hips, and shoulders should be aligned.
> • Each side of the body should carry an equal amount of weight.
> • The muscles should be relaxed.

obsessive about what you eat, or about the amount of exercise you try to do. Set yourself realistic targets, ones that you know you can achieve. If you find it difficult to begin with, make up a chart and monitor your daily progress, marking down how many push-ups or kickbacks you managed on a particular day, and then try increasing them the following day, but do it gradually.

Most importantly, do remember—whatever stage you are at—to think positively and keep visualizing your goal as you work through each movement. There's that fit, healthy, and confident new you out there, either waiting to be discovered or anxious to be maintained!

warming up

The warm-up exercises will help you release any tension held in the mind or body before you start on your exercise session. They will also mobilize and stretch all the muscles in preparation for the more demanding exercises. It is essential to do these warm-ups, whether you will then be moving on to the Introductory or Advanced level exercises.

Loosening up the body before exercising is important because it prepares the muscles and joints for the workout and also increases the heart rate, causing the blood to pump faster around the body. Consequently, the harder the muscles work, the more beneficial the exercise will be. Warm-up exercises should be a blend of rhythmic stretching so that all parts of the body are limbered up and ready to go.

Each of the five exercise chapters begins with a series of warm-up exercises. The idea is that you choose a couple of the exercises shown and allow for time to warm up thoroughly. You can alternate the warm-ups from one session to the next so you don't get bored. Ideally, the routine should take 5–10 minutes to perform.

Relax, concentrate, and work slowly and steadily, following the instructions precisely. Do not try to push any of the moves too far, too soon—you are making progress the whole time, even if it does not seem that way. Always keep the principles in mind and always think "quality."

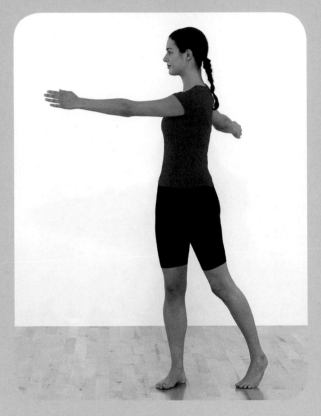

Starting gently

If you are completely new to exercising, you can limit your session to the warm-up exercises only, just for a week or two, so you can really ease into the exercise routine. It is also a good idea to stick to the warm-up movements only for a short while if you have not taken any form of exercise for some time and perhaps feel stiff and inflexible as a result. You may find that this stage is enough of a challenge in itself at first, but in no time at all you will have loosened up your joints and started to improve your muscle tone, and you will feel ready, able, and eager to tackle the next step.

The warm-up exercises are also ideal for mobilizing you first thing in the morning—after all, no self-respecting cat would wake up after a long sleep and start moving about without first having a good stretch in all directions! And they are a quick and effective way to iron out the kinks—both in the body and the mind—that tend to accumulate during a busy working day. Remember, however, that the warm-up exercises are not a "quick fix"—you must always put the full amount of focus and concentration into preparation and execution.

cooling down

Many people dismiss cooling down after exercise as a waste of time or simply unimportant. In reality, the cooldown is just as important as the warm-up if you want to stay injury free. However, while the main purpose of warming-up is to prepare the body and mind for exercising, cooling down and stretching plays a different role.

Just as you need to prepare the body for exercising with warming-up exercises, you also need to cool it down after you have finished. After all, your body has been through quite an ordeal!

The main aim of the cooldown is to promote recovery and return the body to a pre-exercise level and, as long as performed properly, to assist your body in its necessary repair process. As with the warm-ups, each of the five chapters features a series of cooldown exercises. Again, the idea is that you choose a couple of the exercises shown and allow around 10 minutes to stretch and cool down. Your body will thank you for it.

The cooldown will also help with "post-exercise muscle soreness." It does this by allowing the muscles to repair and align themselves after the exercises. This prevents the soreness that is usually experienced the day after a workout, particularly if you haven't done any exercise for a while or if you are a beginner to exercise.

Cooling down and stretching also increases your flexibility, which means you will be able to have a fuller range of movement through your joints.

While most forms of exercise will help you to burn calories and fat while strengthening and defining the muscles, stretching helps to tone and lengthen them. The result is that you can appear slimmer, even if you haven't lost any weight. However, if you practice regularly, the toning effects of stretching can make it easier to lose stubborn pounds and give you a more streamlined silhouette overall. So, you'll be one step closer to fitting into your "skinny" jeans! You may even find that you look taller, because some of the stretches in this section will help you to develop a better posture.

Stretch to relax and detox

If you need any more convincing, you'll be pleased to learn that stretching also has great benefits for the mind. While it does require a degree of concentration, to make sure you're doing each stretch correctly and to the best of your ability, you'll soon realize how relaxing it can be.

Since stretching is best done in silence or to slow and soothing music, it can almost be like meditating. Setting aside just a few minutes at the end of your routine will help to put you in a positive frame of mind for the day to follow.

As you become more familiar with the different stretches, you can combine the movements with deep breathing and positive visualizations, which will help you to clear your mind of clutter.

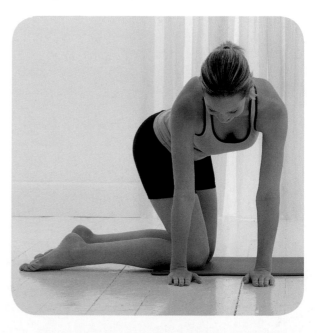

effective exercising

You might be wondering whether a short exercise session each day is enough to make a difference to your body, but the good news is that it works.

The most effective way to burn off excess fat is to work the body aerobically and to learn exercises that will increase muscle and at the same time reduce fat. With a warm-up to start, and a cooldown to finish, the exercise routines in this book are designed to do just that.

We recommend you start with our plan and monitor your results, but only you will know your body's major trouble zones, so you can include extra exercises to target those particular areas. Once you become familiar with the exercises, you can easily draw up your own plan. Make sure you include a good mix to work all the body areas but, if you want to aim for weight loss as well as toning, remember that the standing exercises will burn a lot more calories than the others. Plus, any exercise that targets the legs will create a big calorie expenditure.

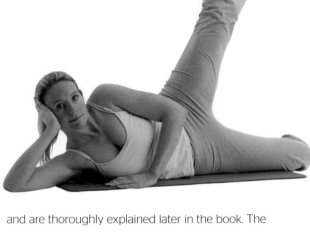

Easy steps

This book divides the main body zones into four chapters, each of which targets a specific trouble area. The sections contain warm-ups, exercises, and cool-down stretches and are thoroughly explained later in the book. The exercises are divided into two levels, introductory and advanced, so you can start your program off at an easy pace, and increase the number of reps as you progress.

These sections are followed by a chapter explaining the benefits of core stability, and includes suggestions and exercises, to help you train your core muscles.

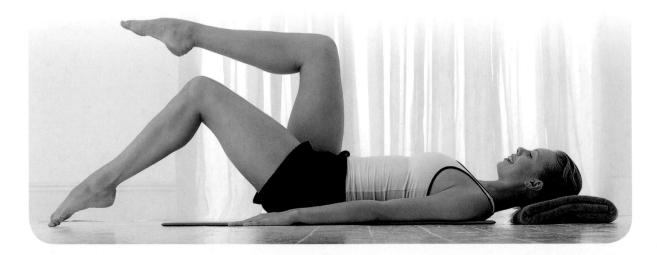

The final chapter contains a 12-week exercise planner that will allow you to work at your own pace, and ultimately achieve your fitness goals.

The planner is organized into two sections, introductory and advanced. The programs clearly list six exercises a day (with page references) that alternate the focus on specific body zones. The final day of the week is a mixture of all the target areas.

Once you've worked through the introductory, or first six-week schedule, and are feeling more confident and fitter, you can progress to the second series of exercises in the advanced plan. It's as easy as that. The plans can be used as an outline guide, so if you find any particular exercises too difficult, feel free to replace them with something else from the same level. However, the closer you stick to the plan we've drawn up, the better you'll find the results will be. Here is a brief insight into what the various areas can help you achieve.

Warming up

Targets: To prepare your muscles ready for exercise.
What's involved: A range of gentle body movements to get the body ready for more strenuous exercises.
Benefits: You need to warm up to avoid injuries.

Exercises

Targets: Each of the major muscle groups in the body—it's an all-over workout.
What's involved: A wide variety of exercises that are fun to do, including standing, sitting, and floor routines.
Benefits: An all-over improvement in muscle tone and shape targeting the whole body.

Cooling down and stretching

Targets: To cool down after an exercise session and to help prevent muscle soreness.
What's involved: A series of stretches that will leave your mind calm and your body more flexible.
Benefits: To help cool your body down, while making your muscles longer, leaner, and more toned.

Exercise plans

Targets: All-over body fitness and toning.
What's involved: An organized series of exercises that start at an easier level and progress through a 12-week plan to achieve all-over fitness.
Benefits: The way to fitness for those new to exercise and looking to progress gradually.

Core stability

Targets: It's an intelligent workout that strengthens your body from the inside out.
What's involved: A series of exercises that will strengthen your core muscles and improve your overall fitness.
Benefits: If your core is strong, your balance and coordination will be improved.

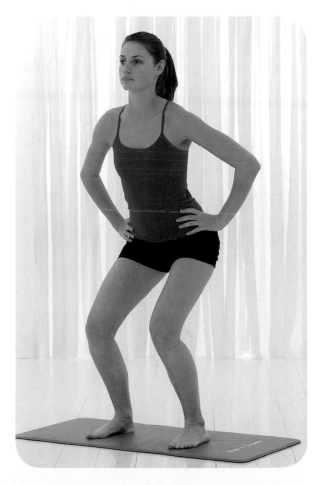

standing posture

Posture is the starting point of all movement. If your posture is under strain, every movement you make will be inefficient, which leads to tiredness, weakness, and aching muscles and joints. This step-by-step process describes how to create a good, stable standing posture that will give you the starting point for more efficient and relaxed movement in all the standing exercises.

How to begin

Stand with your feet pointing forward about hips' width apart, your hands on your hips, and your shoulders as relaxed as possible. It's helpful to stand in front of a mirror, because this will give you a better idea of how you hold yourself. Gradually move your body in circles, then forward and backward, and finally to the left and to the right, to find a central, relaxed point. Then, bring your attention to each area of your body in turn, as described below and on the following pages, to release tension. Notice how each area feels when it is relaxed, then breathe deeply in and out five times before you move on.

As you start to concentrate on the upper body, you may find that the lower areas move out of alignment. Keep checking the areas of the body you have centered and bring them back into good alignment as you continue working upward. The more often you do this exercise, the easier it will get.

Feet

Focus on your feet. Be aware of how your weight is distributed between the insides and outsides, and heels and balls of your feet. Gently sway your body, backward and forward, from side to side, and around in circles, to distribute your weight more evenly.

Calf muscles

Move your attention to your calf muscles and your shins. Again, shift your weight gently in all directions, noticing how the tension builds and relaxes. When you find the most central point, relax into it and breathe deeply in and out five times.

How to check your posture

Stand tall in front of a full-length mirror to assess your posture when you are standing. Check to see whether the following applies:

• Earlobes level • Shoulders level • Kneecaps level
• Equal distance between shoulders and ears
• Equal distance between arms and body • Hips level

Now turn and look at yourself sideways. Imagine there is a straight line drawn down the center of your body. If your posture is correct, the line will pass through the center of the earlobe, the tip of the shoulder, halfway through the chest, slightly behind the hip, and just outside the ankle bone.

Knees

Concentrate on your kneecaps. Do you feel tension or pressure in these areas? If so, shift your weight gently in all directions until you feel the knees release or unlock. Check that the soles of your feet and your calves remain relaxed throughout this stage. Hold this position and take five deep breaths in and out.

Thigh muscles

Many people think that hard thigh muscles have the best kind of tone, but your thighs actually need to be relaxed as well as strong. It can be difficult to release tension from the thighs, so take as much time as you need when working on this area. Shift your weight in circles, backward and forward and from side to side until you feel your thighs relax. Take five breaths and relax.

Pelvis and buttocks

This area is the center of your posture. To find a neutral, relaxed position, first gently and slowly tip your pelvis forward and backward (tucking your tailbone in and out) until you feel the place where there is the least amount of tension. Once you have done this, start shifting your weight from left to right until your pelvis is as central as possible and you feel near-equal pressure on your feet.

This is the neutral pelvis position, which you will be directed to adopt in some of the exercises. Slowly scan up your lower body and check that you are maintaining the releasing feeling in your feet, calves, knees, and thighs. Hold this position and breathe in and out five times.

Stomach wall

Bring your attention to the abdomen. Tighten your stomach muscles as much as possible, then release. Try to find a middle tension between full tightening and total relaxation because this will help you to develop good abdominal muscle tone. In addition, shift your weight gently forward and backward, left and right, and in circles until you feel your abdominals reach the middle point of tension. Hold and breathe in and out five times.

Back

Your lower back is the most vulnerable part of your back. To release tension here, concentrate on relaxing the area between your buttocks and shoulder blades.

First, tuck your tailbone in slowly and at the same time raise your shoulders gently upward. You will feel the tension run along the entire length of your spine. Once you are aware of tension building up, stop and return to your original position.

Now, perform the opposite action. Bring your shoulder blades backward and downward while at the same time raising your tailbone. Again, as soon as you feel tension building, stop and gently return to your starting position. Move gently and slowly between these two actions until you find the point that holds the least tension. Hold this position and breathe deeply in and out five times.

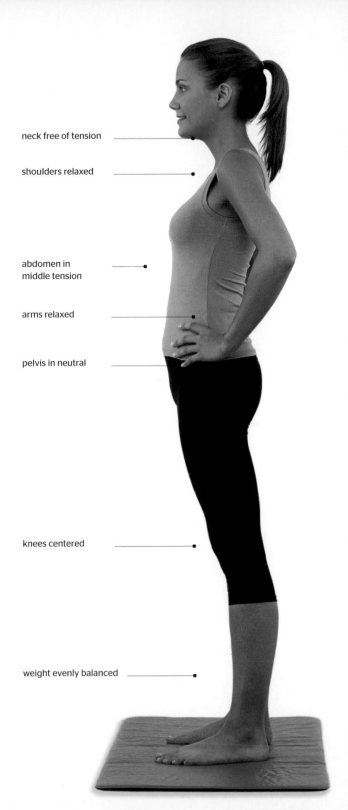

neck free of tension

shoulders relaxed

abdomen in middle tension

arms relaxed

pelvis in neutral

knees centered

weight evenly balanced

Chest

Poor tone in the chest can cause poor posture, which will restrict your breathing. Finding the middle area between deep breathing and shallow breathing and relaxing into it is the objective here. Take some shallow, then some deep breaths, breathing into your back and the sides of your rib cage. Allow your breath to find a middle depth and breathe in and out five times. Take your attention to the feet and work your way up your body, checking you are retaining a relaxed posture. Take five breaths and relax.

Shoulders

Gently pull your shoulders backward and upward as tightly as you are able to without straining. Then, bring your shoulders down and forward. Again, find the middle ground, relax into it, and take five breaths in and out. Take another five breaths and relax.

Arms

Let your arms hang as dead weights and then gently turn them inward and outward. In addition, slowly swing your arms backward and forward to find a tension-free central point. Take five breaths and relax into your posture.

Neck

To find a tension-free position for the neck, use forward-bending, backward-bending, looking-right, and looking-left movements. You can also tip your head sideways to the left and right. Take your time to work between the movements and find a middle point of tension release. Take five breaths, then take your attention to your feet and work your way up the body to ensure your posture is relaxed throughout.

Summary

This is a simple approach to find good posture in a standing position, which you can practice at any time. The tension-release procedures take time and practice to master. However, you should experience a feeling of lightness, as though your body is lifting upward.

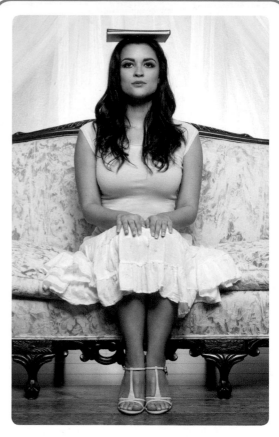

Here are some simple steps to help you to improve your posture:

1. When walking, make a conscious effort to keep your backbone straight and hold your shoulders back. Pull in your stomach and buttocks and tuck in your chin.
2. When seated, sit up straight, do not cross your legs.
3. If working at a desk, choose a seat in which you are comfortable and which is at the correct position for your desk. The seat should be high enough to allow your thighs to rest horizontally on the seat.
4. Wear sensible low-heeled shoes. Keep high ones for the occasional night out. Shoes with low heels put far less strain on your back than stiletto heels.
5. Practice walking around the house with a heavy book balanced on your head, as though you were at a deportment class. The aim is to reach the other end of the room with the book still on your head.

sitting posture

This will encourage you to sit in a good relaxed posture. Most people spend a lot of time sitting but tend to slouch instead of sitting upright. This exercise helps to retrain the body and you can practice it any time you are sitting down.

1 Sit on the front two-thirds of the chair with your feet placed flat on the floor and hips' width apart. (You can sit with your buttocks against the back of the chair if you are practicing this in your daily life but moving forward reduces the temptation to lean back.) Drop your shoulders, place your hands on your thighs, and relax your pelvic floor muscles—the same ones you can use to control the flow or urine. Breathe in deeply and widely, projecting your breath into your back and the sides of your rib cage. Elevate up slightly through your spine to help straighten your posture.

2 Breathe out with control, tightening the muscles of your pelvic floor to about 50 percent of your tension potential. Breathe in and release the tension in your pelvic floor, then breathe out and tighten your pelvic floor just short of full tension. Breathe in again and release the tension, then breathe out, this time tightening your pelvic floor muscles to near-capacity tension. Breathe in and then out, then relax. Rest for 30–60 seconds. Repeat three times.

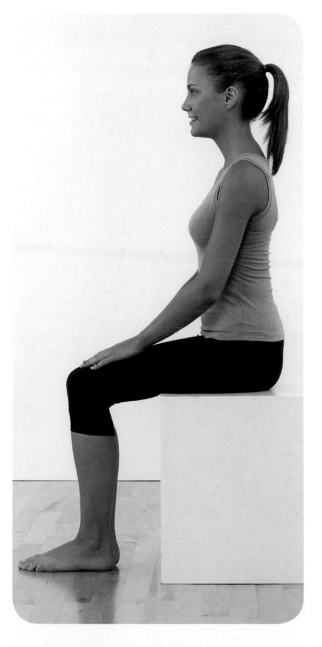

> **Safety points**
> • You want your spine to be erect without forcing it.
> • Do not hold this position for too long the first few times that you try it. It may take time for you to feel comfortable in a good sitting posture.

you and your body

Before you embark on an exercise routine, it is very helpful to have a basic understanding of how your body works, and why it's important to be aware of your current level of fitness before you start. Being muscle aware will help you target the areas you want to firm up.

How your body moves

Your body's framework is the skeleton, made up of more than 200 bones that support your body and allow you to move. Muscles attached to the ends of bones permit an enormous range of movement. However, joints and muscles that aren't regularly exercised become stiff and immobile, leading to pain and possible injury.

Muscles are made up of millions of tiny protein filaments that relax and contract to produce movement. Most muscles are attached to bones by tendons and are consciously controlled by your brain. Movement happens when muscles pull on tendons, which move the bones at the joints.

Most movements require the use of several muscle groups. They should be loaded with resistance, and

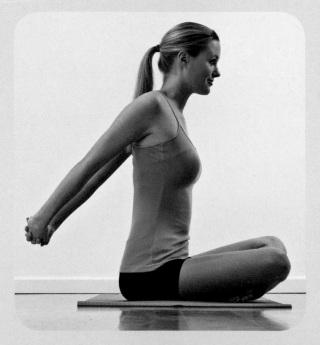

challenged in a variety of ways—by lateral (side) flexion, bending forward and backward, and rotation. If strength and muscle toning is the goal; hundreds of repetitions are not necessary. Your strength should be developed gradually to decrease the risk of injury. When starting out on a training program, you need to progress properly:
• Start with the easiest movements and progress to more difficult movements.
• Perform all movements in a slow and controlled manner until coordination, strength, and confidence permit higher-speed movements.

Why toned muscles look so much better

Looking good and feeling good go hand in hand, so if you are conscious of your flabby stomach or buttock muscles, it will do little to boost your self-confidence and make you feel good about yourself. Time invested in dealing with the problem will change your whole outlook on life:
• you will look good in whatever clothes you wear
• your confidence in yourself will soar
• your posture will be improved
• you will not have back discomfort.

Basic rules when exercising

Whatever your age, before exercising it is important to remember these basic guidelines.
• Exercise at a rate that feels right for you.
• Don't exercise when you feel unwell.
• Always warm up and cool down to prevent injury.
• Don't push yourself too hard—build up gradually.
• Check with your doctor if you have any medical condition, especially if you are pregnant.

Pregnancy

Pregnancy is not an illness. As long as you feel well, can still move around easily and the growing baby is not in the way there is no reason to stop exercising. If you have doubts, seek medical advice.

Minor illnesses

As with any other form of exercise, do not attempt to work off any minor illness while exercising. This is especially important in cases of viral chest, throat, influenza, and glandular infections, which affect your muscular system. Make sure you have been free from symptoms for at least two weeks.

Assessing your level of fitness

Before you get started with an exercise program, it's advisable to think about and assess your current level of fitness. It's possible to do this on your own, but getting advice from a medical expert or fitness instructor can also be valuable.

If you are new to exercising, have not exercised for a while, or have had or have a medical problem, it's advisable to see a doctor before you embark on a fitness routine. Book an appointment for a medical checkup and to discuss your health. Apart from ensuring that your health is currently good and that you don't have any issues you're unaware of, this will also provide you with the reassurance that you can start exercising without expecting any problems. Once you've been given the all clear, you can decide on where to start and identify your initial goals.

Your resting heart rate

As well as getting checked over by a medical professional, one of the best and easiest ways of establishing how fit you are is to find out what your resting heart rate is. To do this, you need to take your pulse when you're not doing exercise. First thing in the morning, when you've just woken up but haven't properly got up, is an ideal time.

Resting heart rate

Take your pulse by either placing two fingers on your neck, just below your jawbone, or on your wrist. Use a stopwatch or watch and count the number of times your pulse beats over ten seconds. Multiply this figure by six to calculate the number of times your pulse beats over a minute. The figure you have is your resting heart rate. For most people, this figure lies between 60 and 80, but the fitter you become and the stronger your heart gets, the lower your resting heart rate will be. Everyone's resting heart rate differs—some forms of medication can increase it and it will tend to be higher if you're unfit or haven't exercised for a while. If you are concerned about the reading you get, speak to your doctor.

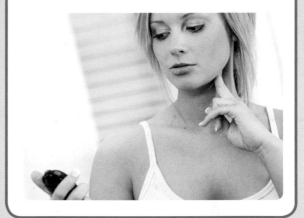

Your resting heart rate may increase naturally as you get older. If it appears to get higher suddenly, after a period of extensive training, this may be an indication that you're pushing yourself too hard and need to slow down your pace or reduce the frequency of your exercising.

Gym assessment

If you are concerned in any way regarding your current fitness, another way to establish how fit you are is to undergo a fitness check with an instructor at a local gym. This can provide a useful overview of your current fitness level and highlight any areas that need particular work.

body types

Although we are all different, people generally fall into one of three basic body types—endomorph, mesomorph, or ectomorph. Not everyone fits exactly into one type, and you may combine elements of two, but there are likely to be qualities of one type that are predominant. Finding out which body type best describes us can be helpful, because each body type has its own characteristics and ways it responds to exercise and diet.

Working with your body shape

We all have a unique bone structure and body shape that, frankly, we can't change. Some of us are genetically programmed to be very slender (ectomorphs), others are curvaceous with a tendency to gain weight (endomorphs), while others tend to be athletic (mesomorphs). It's important to work out the shape you are before embarking on your fitness routine—if you are a natural endomorph, no amount of exercise or dieting will give you a waiflike, ectomorphic look. Furthermore, women are naturally designed to store fat on the hips and thighs to protect the reproductive organs—that is, until the menopause, after which they will store fat around the midsection.

Endomorph

If you are an endomorph, your body will tend to be pear-shaped, so that your hips are broader than your shoulders and you have a wide bone structure. You're also more likely to have a curvier body than other types, and may be prone to gaining weight and storing fat. Various forms of aerobic activity are good methods for controlling this.

Mesomorph

If you are a mesomorph, then you're likely to be of average weight—neither plump nor skinny—and have a shape that falls somewhere between endomorph and

Apples and pears

Use the following technique to discover whether you're more of an apple than a pear. You're apple-shaped if the ratio is 0.8 or more for women and 1.0 or more for men. If the ratio is less than 0.8 or 1.0, you have more of a pear shape (endomorph).

1. Place a tape measure directly onto your skin (not over clothes) and measure your waist at the navel and your hips at their widest point.

2. To work out your waist to hip ratio, divide the waist measurement by the hip measurement. The result will be your waist to hip ratio.

Of course, you may have a neutral body shape that's neither apple or pearlike. If this sounds like you, then stick to a good exercise routine, eat a healthy balanced diet, and enjoy your choice of training.

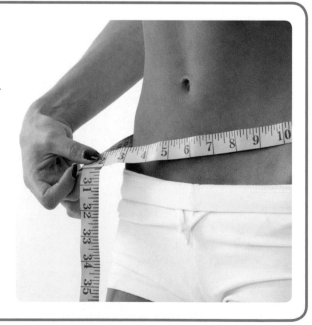

ectomorph. Your shoulders may be wider than your hips and you may have a tendency to gain muscle quite easily, but you'll generally have little in the way of body fat. You'll also find it relatively easy to lose weight. A balanced exercise program that perhaps includes some aerobic activities (see following page) is a good option for mesomorphs, because it will ensure the whole body is being exercised.

Ectomorph

Typical ectomorphs are thin and have a small frame. Your shoulders and hips will be narrow, you'll have very little in the way of body fat, and a narrow chest and stomach. Your legs and arms will also be thin and you will have a narrow face with a high forehead.

Ectomorphs tend to flourish with exercise. However, this body type can be prone to fatigue and it's important not to attempt too much when you're tired.

Apple and pear

You may have come across the terms apple and pear to describe body shapes. If you're an apple, then you tend to gain fat in the midsection of the body—the stomach, chest, and abdomen.

People with pear-shaped bodies tend to store fat below the waistline. Although it's regarded as healthier to be pear-shaped than apple-shaped, the thighs, buttocks, and hips may need extra attention to keep them in shape. The cooldown and stretching exercises that focus on these areas will be doubly important.

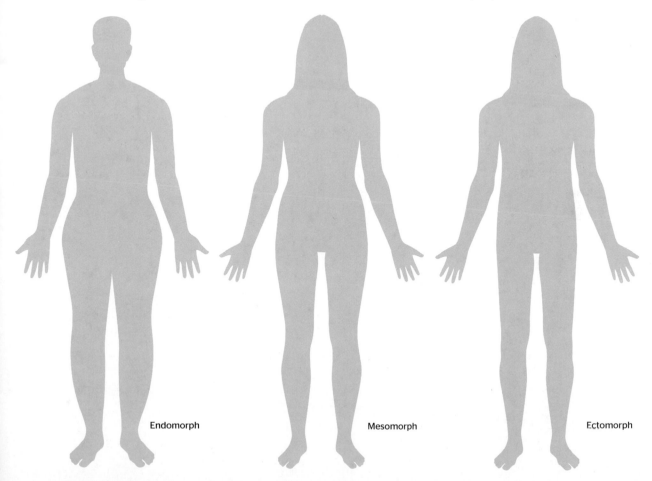

Endomorph   Mesomorph   Ectomorph

other fitness options

If you want to get fit, then you'll have to include some activity that raises your heartbeat for at least 15 minutes at a time. There are two main types of exercise that will help you achieve fitness. One is aerobic exercise and the other is toning or strengthening work.

Both are important, but if the concept of donning a leotard and taking up step aerobics at the local gym fills you with horror, or the mere mention of jogging causes an outbreak of athlete's foot, relax—there are plenty of other options!

Aerobic exercises

These exercises help to burn fat and involve any form of activity that makes you feel a little out of breath. They include: cycling, jogging, skipping, power walking, running, and swimming.

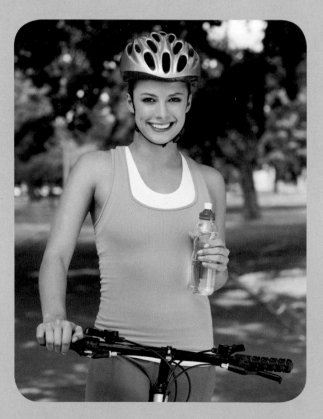

Toning or strengthening exercises

These exercises, such as the ones in this book, build up specific muscle groups and, in doing so, increase the rate at which the calories you take in are used up.

Cycling

The idea of squeezing into a pair of Lycra shorts and hitting the highways on your bike may not fill you with an adrenalin rush but when you consider its health benefits, it is well worth a second thought.

Cycling is an ideal exercise for toning up muscles, getting out in the fresh air, and just dashing out to the store. If you're new to cycling, it's important to begin slowly and not overdo it, even if you consider yourself to have a good fitness level. Each sport differs and requires a different set of skills and the use of a specific range of muscles, so being fit in one sport doesn't necessarily mean you'll slip with ease into another. The bike you use should be comfortable, in safe working order, and the right size for your height.

When you first begin, start out slowly by doing short rides on the bike, for example 20–25 minutes at a time. As you get used to cycling and build up your cycling fitness level, you can increase the time.

Water aerobics

This is based on normal aerobic exercises such as running, jogging, and walking, but the exercises are performed in water, generally at a local swimming pool. It is a perfect form of all-round exercise and the idea is to work the muscles against the resistance of the water while keeping an upright stance throughout the exercise sequence. It is a great way of burning up calories efficiently.

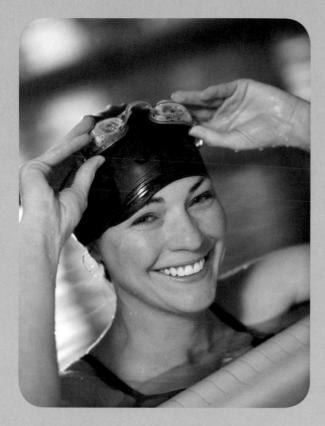

Power walking

How about taking up power walking? Not a gentle saunter around the park but a brisk walk, head and shoulders back, arms swinging, stomach held in, and taking long determined strides. Not only will it encourage better posture, but power walking is also ideal for toning up the thighs, arms, and legs. The more intense you make it, the more calories you will burn up. And when you are powering along, make sure that you take in deep breaths of fresh air.

Exercising for new mothers

After giving birth, some women are devastated to find themselves left with saggy stomach muscles and a bigger backside. While other parts of the body slowly get back into shape, these areas often seem reluctant to return to their former size.

Don't worry—with some gentle exercising, that flab will soon disappear and you will be able to climb into those clinging denims again.

But before you put on your training clothes and set yourself an exercise schedule to follow, here are a few important rules:

• Check with your doctor about exercising and ask if they can recommend any gentle firming-up exercises. Remember childbirth is a traumatic experience for the body and you cannot expect it to snap back into its previous condition just like that.

• Develop a routine. Wait until the baby is having a nap, or has gone to bed, before you start exercising.

• Make sure that each of your movements is slow and take adequate rest breaks between exercises.

• Warm up and cool down before and after each exercise session.

• If one day you feel under the weather or it is hot, reduce your routine by half, and make sure that you drink plenty of water to prevent dehydration.

• Simply taking the baby out for a walk is good exercise; remember that a happy contented mother makes for a happy contented baby.

Swimming

Swimming is one of the least stressful forms of exercise so it's an ideal choice to complement your exercise program. Plus you don't need to invest in expensive equipment to begin.

Swimming helps stretch the hamstrings and hips, too, and the action of moving your legs in the water can improve flexibility in your ankles. Aim to swim for up to 30 minutes per session; you can increase your time in the water as fitness levels increase.

Some people love swimming, but for those of us who aren't natural swimmers, plowing along at the same pace can become monotonous. Thankfully there are ways of alleviating the boredom. To provide variety, try alternating between different strokes—one lap of front crawl followed by a lap of backstroke and then butterfly. Or try speeding up your pace for one lap, then slowing down for the next.

a healthy diet

"You are what you eat" is one of those irritating platitudes that happens to be true. Stuff yourself with junk food or drink too much alcohol and you will feel tired, bloated and sluggish. Eat a well-balanced diet and you will feel much more alert and full of increased vitality and vigor.

If you turn green with envy every time you see a young model flaunting her well-toned abdomen and beautifully shaped rear end, don't imagine that she achieved her shape without any effort—she'll know that a healthy diet is as important as exercise.

Following the rules

Remember, it doesn't matter how much exercise you do, it can never fully compensate for poor eating habits. The only way to get fit and eliminate surplus fat is:
• Change your eating habits.
• Increase your level of exercise.
By sticking to these two basic rules, you will be well on your way to achieving that perfect shape.

Nourishing the body

Changing eating habits does not mean that you have to follow a diet and count all your calories. What it does mean is that you should eat healthy, nourishing food containing a balance of essential nutrients, which in turn are derived from the following:

Carbohydrates: These provide energy for the body and come in two basic forms. Simple carbohydrates basically comprise sugar and very little else. Complex carbohydrates include starchy foods, such as bread, potatoes, cereal, pasta, and rice.

Fats: The number one enemy in terms of a lean body but essential for helping to insulate and protect the organs and nerves. Fats are found in varying quantities in foods such as butter, cheese, lard, snacks, and fatty meat. The basic principle of a healthy diet is to reduce the amount of fat you eat. It doesn't mean cutting fat out totally, but instead choosing those foods sensibly.

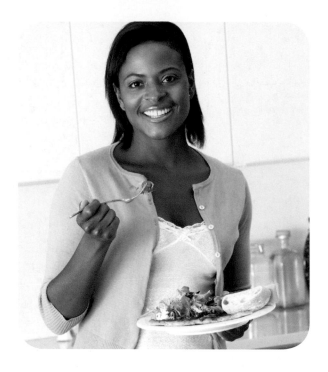

Proteins: The body breaks down the protein from food into its component parts, called amino acids, which it then uses to build and repair tissue and muscle. Protein is found in products such as meat, poultry, fish, dairy foods, eggs, beans, lentils, and nuts.

Minerals: These are vital to the human body because they help to form bones, strengthen teeth, maintain a healthy immune system, and support the vitamins in their work. Calcium, for instance, is important for helping to build strong bones and teeth.

Vitamins: These substances are vital for good health and the maintenance of various bodily functions. A well-balanced diet containing plenty of fresh foods should be rich in vitamins.

Low-fat food

If you follow the advice outlined here, you may have to cut out certain favorite foods, but with such a wide and varied choice remaining for you, that will not seem such a hardship unless you are a veritable slave to cakes and chocolate. All the time you are abstaining, remember the reason that you are doing so.

There are several ways to help cut back the fat content in your food:

- Use low-fat or skim milk.
- Whenever possible, steam, broil or bake food, instead of frying it.
- Use low-fat yogurt instead of cream, ice cream or other dairy products.
- Eat cottage cheese instead of regular fat-filled cheese.
- Add more fish and poultry to your diet.
- Always trim any visible fat off meat.
- Simmer ingredients in vegetable stock instead of shallow frying them in lard or butter.

Of course, you do need a small amount of fat in your diet but, by following these guidelines, you will ensure that you do not get too much.

What to eat

The healthiest diet is one that is high in fruit, vegetables, grains, and beans and low in animal and dairy products. Nutritional guidelines are based on the traditional eating habits of people who live around the Mediterranean, where there is a history of long life expectancy and low rates of heart disease.

- Complex carbohydrates should form half your daily diet.
- Eat at least five portions of fruit and vegetables a day.
- Eat oily fish at least once a week.
- Limit your consumption of red meat and cheeses.
- Eat plenty of fiber-rich foods.
- Reduce your salt intake—use in cooking only.
- Limit your sugar intake—try not to use too much in tea and coffee.
- Eat fresh foods whenever possible and cut back on processed foods.

- Drink alcohol in moderation, and try to have at least two alcohol-free days a week.
- Drink enough fluids to keep your urine pale—at least eight glasses of water a day to flush out toxins. A glass of water every couple of hours will make you feel much more alert.
- Limit your consumption of tea, coffee, cola-type drinks, and chocolate.

When to eat

Optimum nutrition means eating the right foods at the right time, and good health depends on eating regular meals. Breakfast jump-starts the metabolism and boosts blood-sugar levels; if you miss it, you may feel tired and unable to concentrate. Lunch should be the biggest meal of the day because this is when the metabolism is at its most effective. Have a light supper at least two hours before you go to bed because it is hard for the body to digest a large meal at the end of the day.

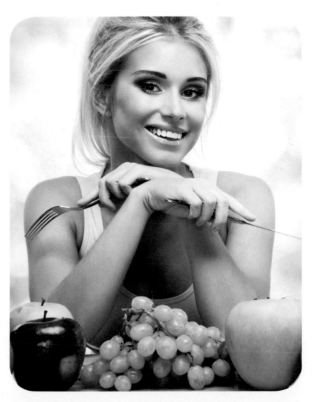

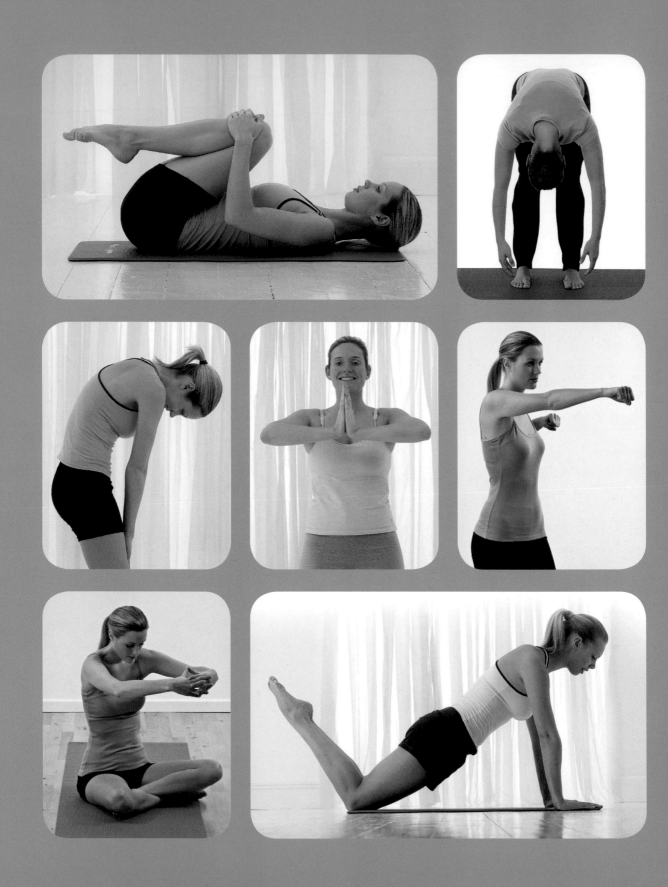

2

chest & back

In this section you will find basic standing and sitting exercises to improve the muscles in the chest and back. Some are traditional exercises or established moves from exercise systems, such as yoga and Pilates, and focus on toning and strengthening exercises for the upper body.

introduction

To keep the chest and back healthy and enable your body to perform a full range of movements, three things are necessary: mobility of the spine, supple muscles, and strength. All these can be achieved by doing moderate exercise regularly and correctly.

The benefits

Doing specific back exercises will help you to ensure that you are working all the important muscle groups. Regular movement helps to maintain the elasticity of the muscles and it builds their power. It also serves to keep the joints mobile. Movement encourages good circulation of blood and other fluids around the body. This helps to keep the joints lubricated and allows muscles and joints to take in nutrients and to expel waste products.

It's important to hold the body correctly when you are exercising and when you are going about your normal day's activities. If the body is held in an abnormal way or you perform an awkward movement, then excessive strain is placed on the joints. This is as true for people who are superfit as it is for those who don't exercise enough. Dancers and yoga practitioners can develop excessive mobility in their joints as a result of performing an outlandish range of movements. This is like driving

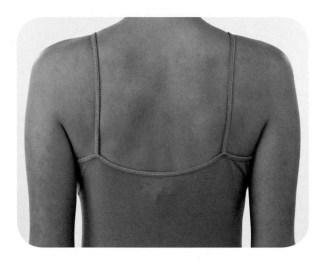

without brakes—the muscles' inbuilt safety mechanisms are not functioning. Mobility needs to be complemented with stability in order to protect the back.

Improving your upper body area

Some women get worried that if they do toning exercises for their upper body they will bulk up. This is simply not true—women do not have enough testosterone to build large muscles. You would have to be lifting heavy weights and following a strict strength-training workout!

Achieving a super-toned body requires a combination of two forms of exercise: the first is toning, as described in this book, and the other is aerobic. The aerobic form of activity will help to burn off any excess body fat as well as improve your cardiovascular health. You should also not forget the importance of eating sensibly, because too many calories in your diet may increase your level of body fat.

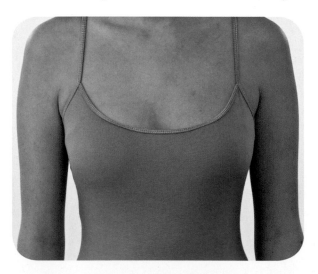

About your upper body muscles

A key to maintaining stability in the upper body is correct use of the deepest abdominal muscle—the transversus abdominis. This muscle is just below your navel and runs in a band from one side of the abdomen to the other. When you contract this muscle, it takes the pressure off the spine. A body builder will instinctively pull in this muscle before lifting a heavy weight.

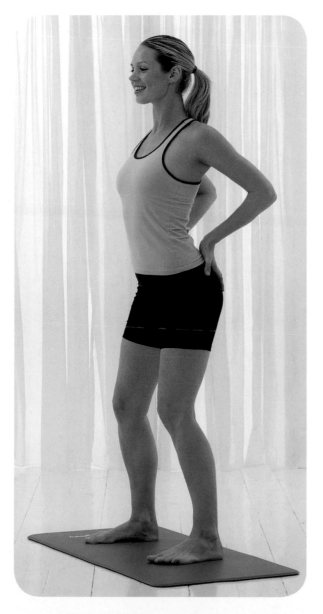

The abdominal muscles work in tandem with the muscles of the back to support and stabilize the spine. When contracted, they increase the pressure in the abdominal cavity, which reduces stress on the spine. Also important are the hip flexors (psoas), which run from the upper part of the thighbone to the lumbar vertebrae, and the hamstrings. Inflexible hip flexors and leg muscles increase the pressure on the back muscles, making back pain or stiffness more likely.

The back muscles

The muscles of the back are arranged in several layers. The superficial muscles, which are closest to the skin's surface, are mainly broad sheets of muscles that connect the vertebrae to the shoulder blades and joints. The middle layer consists of strap-shaped muscles that run over the lower ribs, chest, and lower back. The deepest muscles run from one vertebra to another, helping to keep them in position.

Middle and lower back

The latissimus dorsi is the largest muscle in the upper body and covers the middle and lower back. This muscle is responsible for the downward movements of the upper arm and the inward rotation of your shoulders.

Chest muscles

The pectoralis major is a large, fan-shaped muscle, which has several attachments. One portion fastens to the middle and inner parts of your collarbone, working with the front of your shoulder to move your arms in front, above, and rotate them inward. The other part attaches to your breastbone and ribs—this muscle is activated by moving your arms only in a downward or forward movement of both arms.

What you'll need

For this section, you'll need a chair, a nonslip mat, and a towel. Don't forget to warm up and cool down!

warming-up exercises

It is always essential to warm up before undertaking any form of exercise. Choose a couple of the exercises shown over the next few pages and spend a little time warming up. You should allow around ten minutes for this, and alternate them so you don't get bored.

rolling down

This will mobilize the spine and will benefit the spine, shoulders, and upper body.

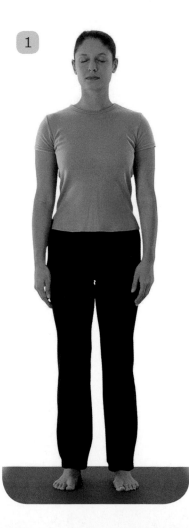

1 Stand upright with your spine in neutral. Place your feet hips' width apart, keep your knees soft, and let your arms hang loosely by your sides.

2 Gently nod your chin toward your chest, then roll forward, keeping the rib cage soft and rolling toward the hips. Sense each vertebra rolling, one at a time.

3 Only roll down to your point of comfort—do not try to go too far too soon. At the bottom of the move, inhale, feeling the air inflate your spine, and keeping the pelvic floor muscles and abdominals engaged.

4 Roll back up, nice and gently. As you finish the roll, exhale and release the shoulder blades. At first, do the roll five times, increasing to a maximum of ten.

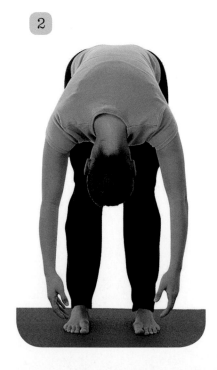

c-curve warm-up

This exercise will help to mobilize the spine and strengthen the central and back muscles.

1 Sit on the floor, with your knees bent, your weight evenly distributed.

2 Place your hands lightly behind your knees, but do not pull on your hands as you carry out the move.

3 Exhale, and rock backward off the pelvis toward the floor.

4 Pause, inhale, and return to the upright start position. Keep the abdominals scooped and hollowed throughout the whole move for support. Only go as far as you can each time without lifting your feet off the floor. Repeat the movement five times, increasing to a maximum of ten.

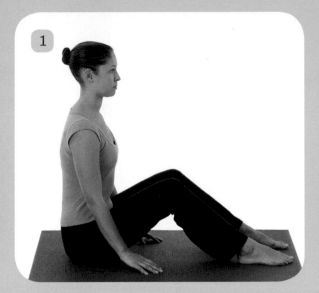

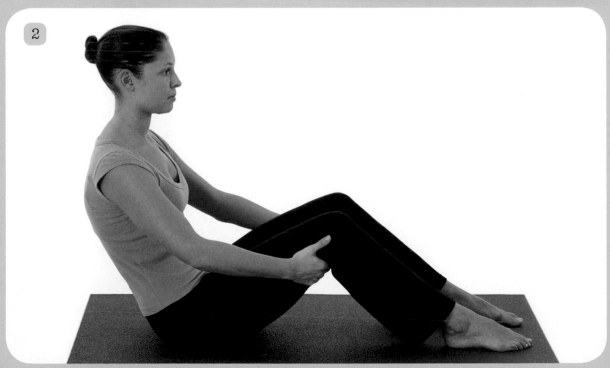

pivot

This mobilizes the whole body and promotes coordination.

1 Stand upright with your spine in neutral. Place your feet wider than hips' width apart, keep your knees soft, and let your arms hang loosely by your sides. Inhale.

2 Exhale, and twist your body to one side. Let your arms swing loosely, moving with you. Your legs will also twist with the movement.

3 Inhale and slowly twist back to the center, exhale and twist to the other side, and then inhale and twist back to the center.

4 Each time you twist, raise your arms higher, until they reach over your head, then work them back down to your sides in a continuous, flowing movement. Take three twists in each direction to get to the top of the movement, and three more twists in each direction to get back down.

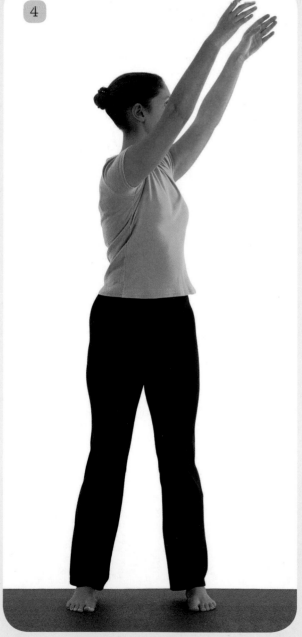

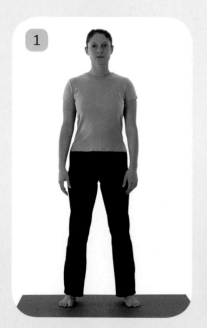

back twists

Gentle back twists from a standing position are easy to control; it is hard to push yourself too far. They give the spine a satisfying stretch, rotating the vertebrae and working the muscles of the back.

1 Stand tall, with your feet hip-width apart. Put your hands on your hips.

2 Slowly turn to the right as far as you comfortably can. Start the turn from the hips, lifting the spine upward as you turn. Keep the neck and head in line with the spine—don't try to turn the head farther because this will put pressure on the neck. Hold the twist for a few moments, breathing normally.

3 Slowly turn back to the center. Then repeat on the other side.

PAY ATTENTION
Try to coordinate your breathing with the movement. Take a deep breath in before you turn, then twist as you breathe out. Return to the center on an out breath, too. This helps you to control the movement.

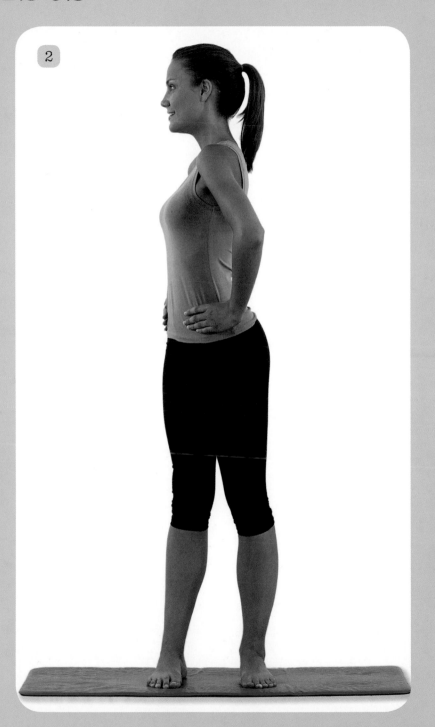

introductory exercises

These first-stage exercises are aimed at beginners, so you should find them relatively easy to start with, allowing you to become more involved as you progress. If you find any of the exercises a bit too difficult, feel free to replace them with something else of the same level.

easy plank (tension hold)

Holding your body in a three-quarters plank shape strengthens the deep transverse muscles that cross the stomach area. Keeping your knees on the floor makes this exercise much easier than the traditional plank, which you can progress to during the advanced exercises.

1 Adopt a traditional push-up position but keep your knees on the floor and your feet in the air. Your fingers should point forward, your elbows stay straight but not locked, your head should be in line with your body, and your feet should be together.

2 Keep your shoulder blades drawn into your back and make sure you don't dip in the middle or raise your backside in the air. Hold this position for a count of ten, breathing regularly throughout.

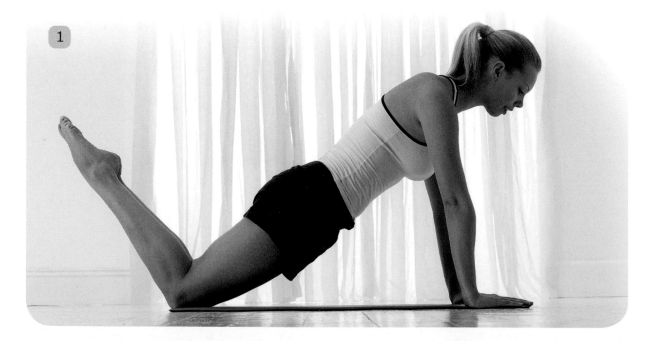

c-curve

This is a progression of the warm-up exercise. This time, position your hands lightly on the sides of your knees. Try to unroll farther each time you practice the movement but only go as far as you can comfortably.

1 Sit on the floor, with your weight evenly distributed and your spine in neutral. Relax your shoulders, with the shoulder blades melting down your back.

2 Inhale, and with the points of your toes gently touching the floor, slowly roll backward off the pelvis. Rock slightly back and forth.

3 Balancing on your toes, inhale as you roll back to the start position.

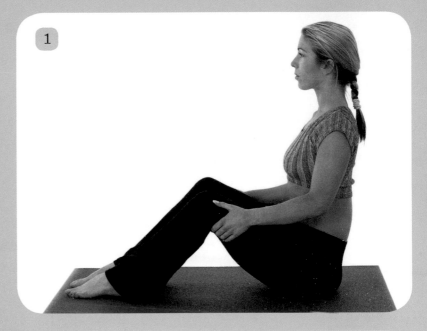

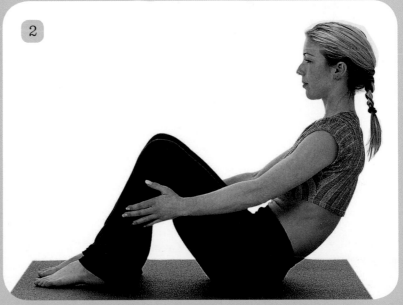

Modification
Relax your feet and lift your toes, resting only your heels on the floor (this will take the tension out of your hip flexors).

standing wall push-up

This exercise is a fantastic way to build upper body strength as well as tone through the back of your upper arm muscles and into your chest.

1 Stand at arms' length away from a wall, with your feet shoulders' width apart. Place your hands against the wall, with your arms stretched out in front of you and your fingers pointing to the ceiling.

2 Keeping your back straight and your head looking straight in front of you, slowly bend your arms at the elbows.

3 Aim to lower yourself a little way toward the wall and then push back to your start position.

PAY ATTENTION

If you want to increase the level of difficulty, try moving your legs farther back. Also, keeping your abdominal muscles pulled in will help tone your stomach muscles.

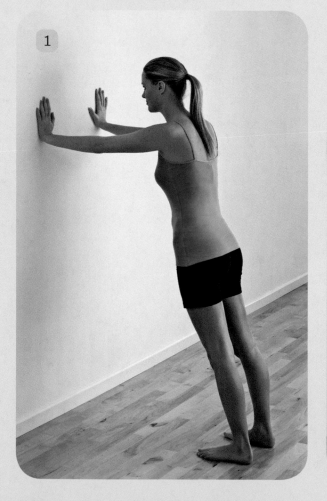

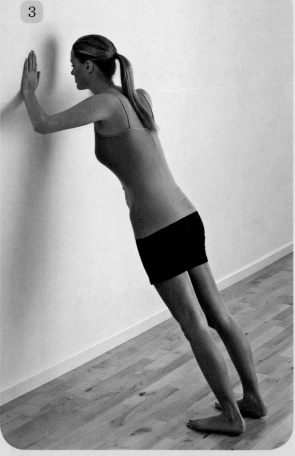

back arch

This exercise helps to stretch the spine backward, countering the effects of slouching. Go only as far as feels comfortable.

1 Lie down on your front. Keep your legs together, tuck your toes under, and place your hands just under your shoulders (as if you were preparing to do a push-up).

2 Very slowly straighten your arms, lifting your head and shoulders upward. Breathe in as you do so. Hold the position for a count of five, breathing, then slowly lower yourself back down.

3 As you repeat the exercise, you may find that you can go a little farther each time. However, do not try to force your back up.

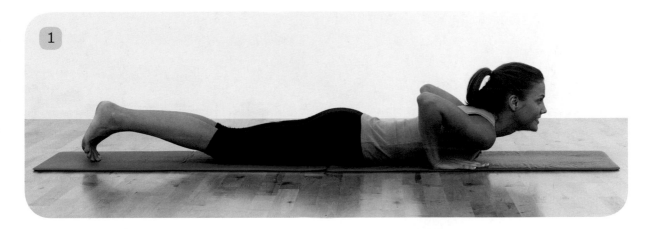

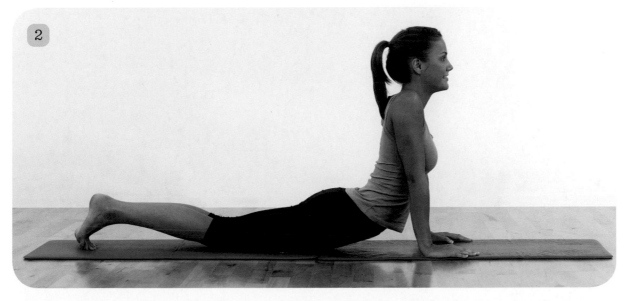

bust lift

This exercise targets the chest muscle, which is responsible for supporting the bust. If this muscle is not exercised, it will become less supportive, which means the bust begins to droop. This is a great way of toning and giving yourself a bust lift.

1 Stand upright with good posture, knees slightly bent, feet hip-width distance apart, and stomach pulled in.

2 Extend your arms out in front of you at chest height, bend the elbows, and join the hands by the palms facing into each other.

3 Stay in this position, press into your palms, and, holding this squeeze, slowly lift your palms a little bit higher. Hold for a second while still applying the squeeze, then slowly lower to the start position, release the squeeze for a second, then reapply and lift.

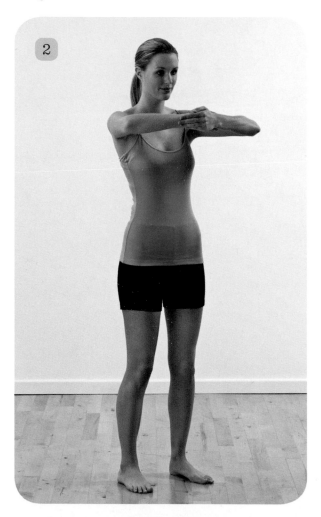

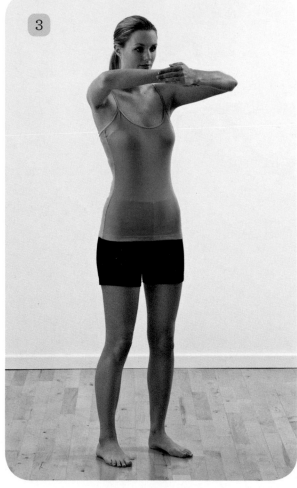

bell pull

This exercise works on toning your arms through your biceps and triceps as well as toning your chest muscle. This is great for women because it helps lift and tone the bust as well as giving the arms a fabulous workout.

1 Stand with good posture, knees slightly bent, and your feet hips' width apart.

2 Lift your arms to shoulder height and then bend at the elbows, so your arms form an L-shape. Press your arms together and keep elbows at shoulder height.

3 Take a deep breath in and then, as you breathe out, gently lift your arms a little bit higher, hold for a second, then lower slowly again. Do all your repetitions on one arm and then repeat on the other arm.

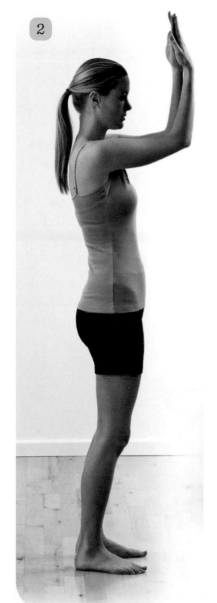

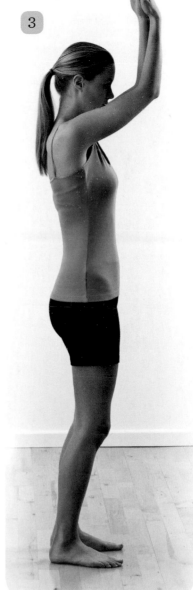

PAY ATTENTION

To get your abdominal muscles working, make sure you keep your stomach pulled in tight to your spine. Also, be sure not to arch your back.

crisscross arms

This simple exercise tones your triceps, biceps, and chest muscles.

1 Sit with good posture, arms extended out in front of you, palms facing each other.

2 Cross your right arm over the left, turning your palms down along the way. Pause, then return to the starting position.

3 Do all your repetitions on one arm and repeat on the other arm.

> ### PAY ATTENTION
> Focus on keeping your abdominal muscles pulled in throughout. To make this more of a challenge, try using weights.

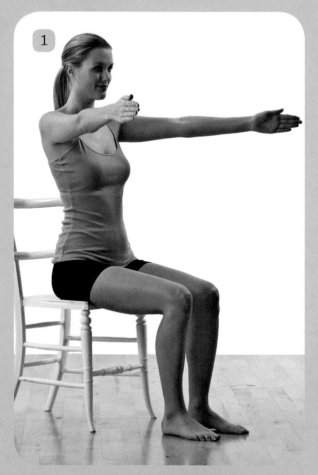

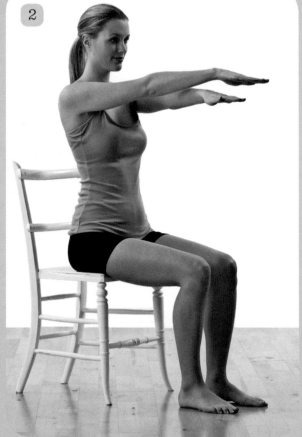

prayer

This is excellent for toning the pectoral muscles (the pecs). Toning these muscles will help to give you a more youthful-looking bust.

1 Either while standing or sitting, press the palms of your hands together at shoulder height while extending your elbows out to the sides.

2 Hold the pose for as long as you can—ideally around ten seconds, pressing your palms together with as much force as you feel comfortable with. Take one second to rest and then repeat the pose.

3 Aim to hold the pose for ten seconds and then take one second to rest and start again.

PAY ATTENTION

Many people will find their joints crack when doing this exercise, so start by pressing the palms lightly together and gradually start to build up the pressure. Doing the exercise this way will help prevent you from getting a cramp.

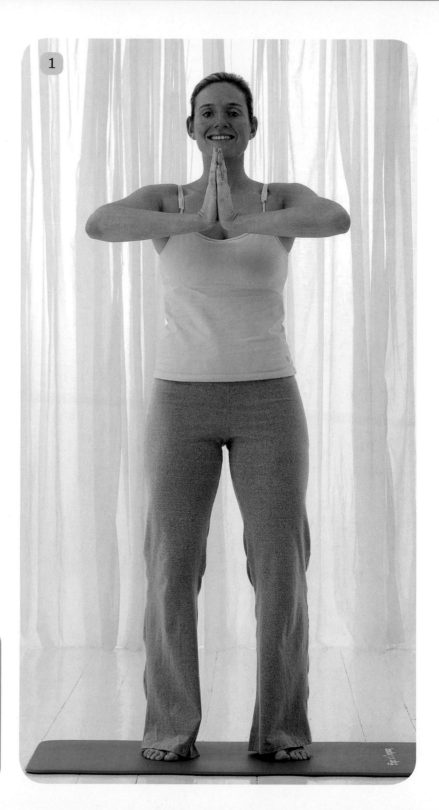

1

easy chest flex

This exercise targets the pectoral muscles, sometimes known as the "pecs," which are the major muscles at the front of the chest. It will also give your supraspinatus muscle, which runs along the top of your shoulder blades, a nice big stretch.

1 You can either stand with feet hips' width apart, or you can do this exercise while sitting on a chair. Whichever position you prefer, make sure that your back is straight and your head and neck are in line with your spine.

2 Bring your arms up to shoulder level and bend from the elbows so that your hands are hovering in front of your chest. Make loose fists with your hands.

3 Leading from the elbow, gently rotate both arms backward so that you're squeezing your shoulder blades together. Your chest will automatically push out a little.

4 Hold for ten seconds, then release.

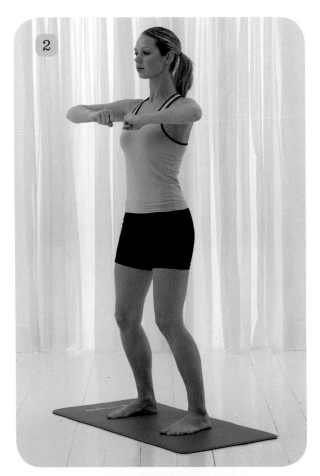

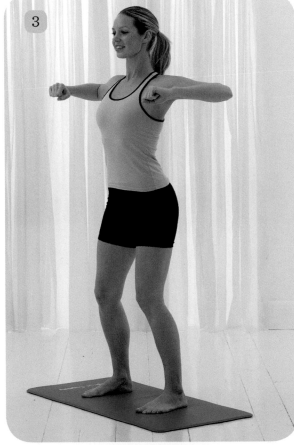

boxing

This is a really fun exercise that will tone your chest, shoulders, and arms. When an exercise works several muscles at once, it increases the amount of calories you burn, both during and after the exercise.

1 Stand up straight with your feet shoulders' width apart, stomach pulled in, and your knees soft, slightly bent.

2 Hold your hands level against your upper chest with both your fists clenched and palms facing inward.

3 Punch one arm forward under control, with your knuckles facing forward. Make sure your hands are level and kept at shoulder height.

4 Bring your hand back to the start position, slowly and under control, and then punch forward with the opposite arm.

> **PAY ATTENTION**
> Keep your knees soft and your stomach pulled in. This will not only work your stomach muscles but will also protect your back.

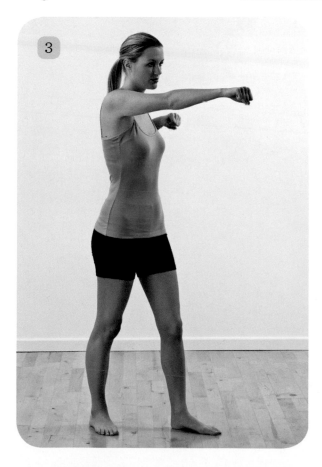

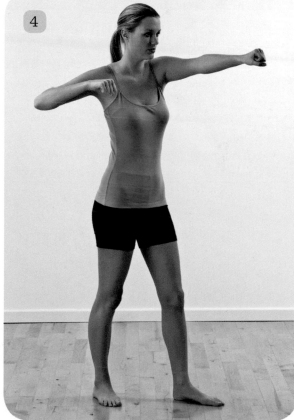

open flyer

This floor exercise will tone through your chest, shoulders, and arms while working on your upper body strength and flexibility.

1 Lie on the mat. Hold a weight in each hand over your chest with your arms up and your palms facing each other.

2 Keeping your elbows slightly bent, lower your arms out to the sides and down until they're level with your chest.

3 Keep your elbows in a fixed position and avoid lowering the weights too low.

4 Squeeze your chest to bring your arms back up, as though you're hugging a tree.

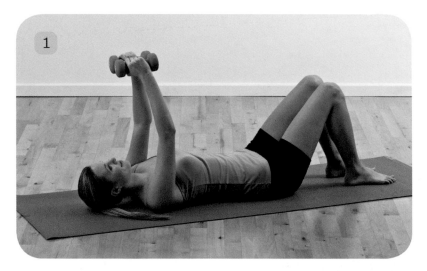

> **PAY ATTENTION**
>
> The slower you perform this exercise, the more effective it is.

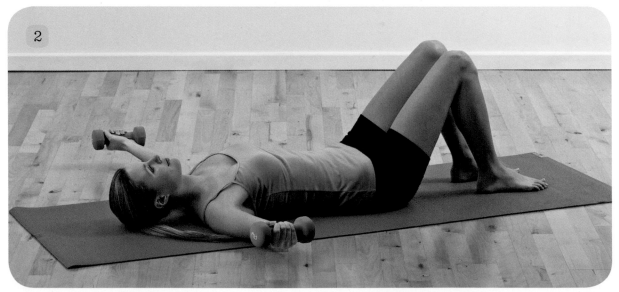

54

front-lying chest lift

The front-lying chest lift is usually used as part of a yoga pose. It's great for stretching out all the muscles across the chest, including the pecs.

1 Lie face down on the floor with your palms on the floor either side of your chest and your legs stretched out behind you.

2 Keeping your hips and thighs on the floor, push up with your hands and arms so that your chest is off the floor. Don't come up too far—aim to lift your chest just a short distance off the floor.

3 Hold the pose for ten seconds, then release and return to the starting position.

> **PAY ATTENTION**
> Some of you may find it hard to arch the back as you lift yourself up into the pose—it depends how flexible you already are. If you can't lift your chest far off the floor, don't abandon this stretch—it will get easier with time.

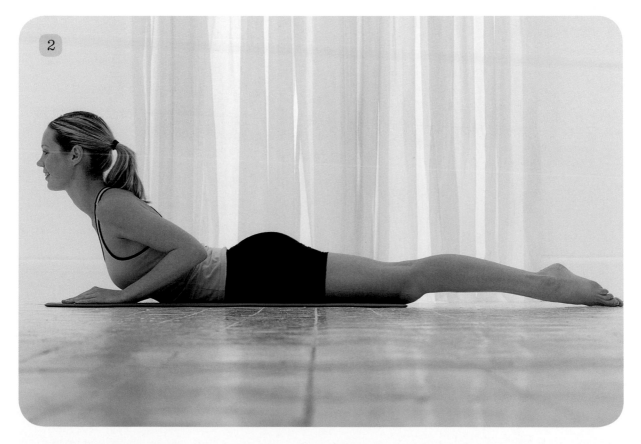

moy complex

This exercise is also known as the "row, rotate, and press" and is a great way to tone the muscles in your back, without having to use the complicated machinery that you find in the gym.

1 Sit on the edge of a chair with a dumbbell or can of soup in each hand.

2 Bend over from the waist so your chest is resting on your knees. Make sure your head and neck are relaxed, so that you're looking down toward the floor.

3 Start with your hands resting on the floor, with elbows slightly bent, then bend your arms and bring your hands up to shoulder level.

4 Rotate your wrists and extend your arms out in front of you so that they're parallel to the floor.

5 Retrace your steps so you're back in the Step 2 position, then repeat the movement.

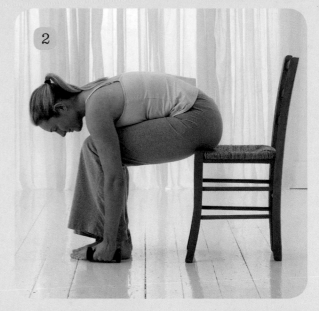

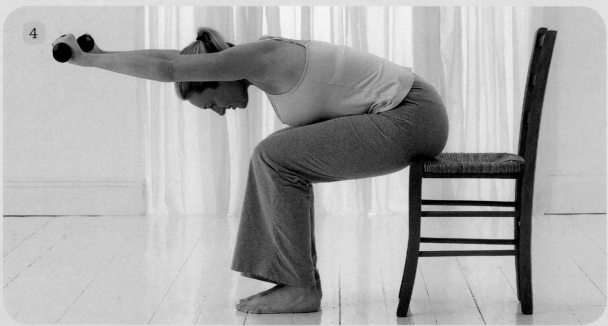

bent-over arm shaper

This sitting exercise will target your arms and your upper back muscles and improve your upper body flexibility and posture.

1 With a weight in each hand, sit on the edge of your chair, bent over, with arms hanging down, feet slightly apart.

2 Keep your abdominal muscles pulled in to stop you from collapsing your back onto your legs.

3 Lift your arms out to the sides, up to shoulder level, squeezing your shoulder blades together.

4 Keep the elbows slightly bent and only lift to your shoulders. Lower the arms and repeat.

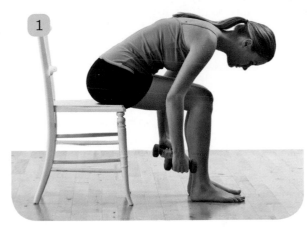

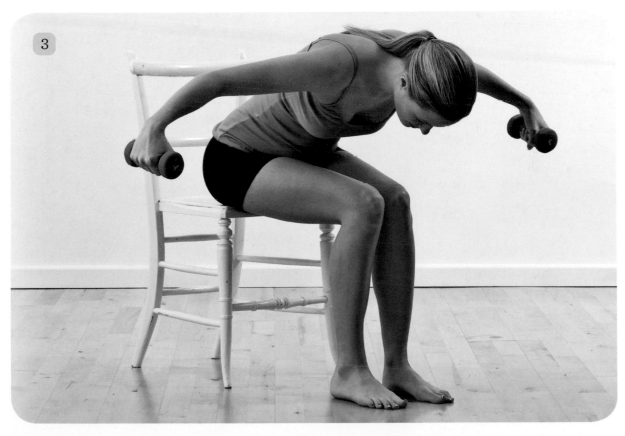

dumbbell row

Doing this exercise is like starting a lawn mower. It targets the muscles in the middle of the back, such as the trapezius. So, if you practice this religiously, it will make wearing backless dresses all the more appealing.

1 Rest your right knee and your right hand on the seat of a chair.

2 Holding a dumbbell or can of soup in your left hand, pull it back toward your hip.

3 Extend your left arm diagonally out in front of you, so it travels toward the ground.

4 Bring the dumbbell back to your hip and repeat the movement.

PAY ATTENTION

You should do this exercise on one side at a time if you have a bad back. If you want to work both sides at once, take away the chair and stand in a squat position while doing the exercise.

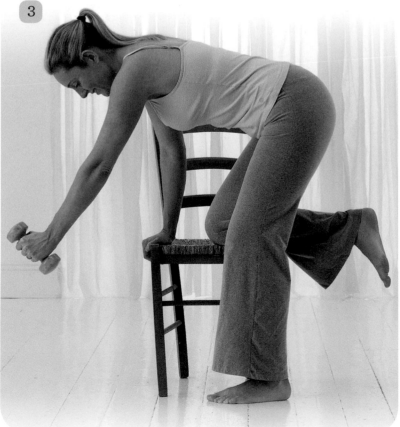

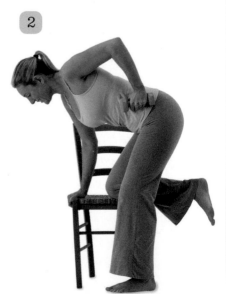

chest press

This exercise targets your triceps and your chest muscle. This is a great exercise for women, because it tightens the muscles that support your bust, giving you a good bust lift.

1 Stand with good upright posture, knees soft, and your feet hips' width apart.

2 Using a weight in each hand, bend your arms so your hands are in front of your shoulders.

3 Gently extend your arms straight out, keeping them at shoulder height.

4 Hold for a second when your arms are fully extended. Slowly return your arms to the start position.

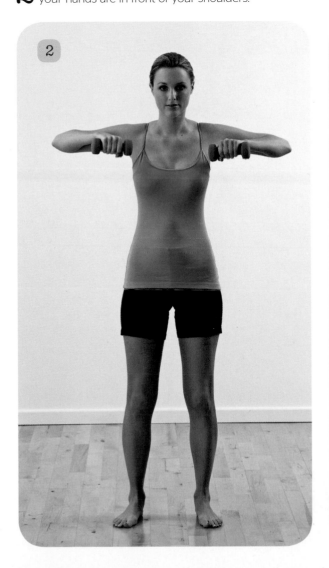

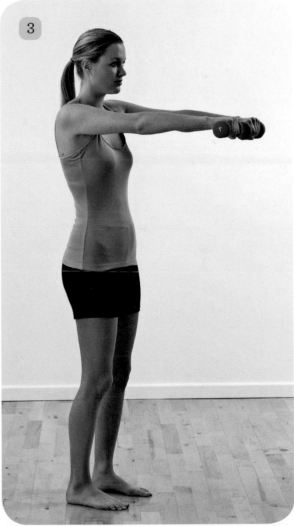

reverse sit-up

This is a great exercise for strengthening the lower back. Adding an arm rotation to the move delivers a double toning boost to the shoulders.

1 Lie flat and face down on the floor with your forehead resting on the backs of your hands.

2 Squeeze your buttocks and use your stomach muscles to raise your chest off the floor as far as you feel comfortable.

3 Squeeze your shoulder blades together by rotating your arms around from the shoulders so your palms are facing downward and your forearms are hovering at chest level.

4 Return your arms to the starting position and lower your chest back down to the floor. Repeat the movement.

PAY ATTENTION

Don't try to pull your chest back too far or it will force your lower back to arch and put a strain on the muscles. Just do what feels comfortable.

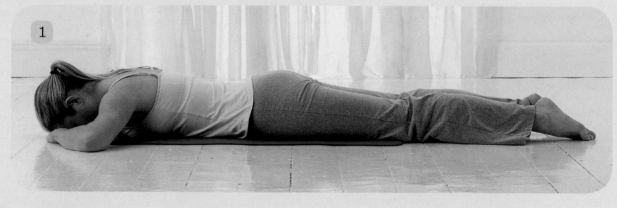

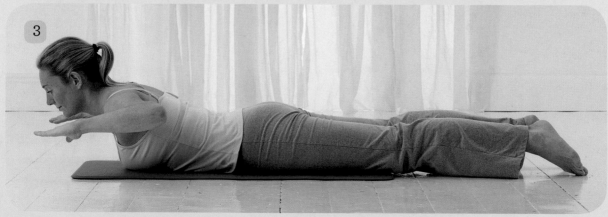

soup-can press

This exercise is great for toning the muscles in your chest and around your collarbone. Make it a priority if you're aiming to squeeze into a strapless dress in a few weeks.

1 Lie on your back, with your knees bent and feet flat on the floor, holding a dumbbell or can of soup in each hand.

2 Bend your elbows and rest your hands by your armpits, so they're hovering just above your shoulders.

3 Extend your arms into the air at a right angle to your body, holding the dumbbells directly over your shoulders with your palms facing away from you.

4 Pull in your abdominals and tilt your chin toward your chest.

5 Release your chin, then bend your elbows and bring your hands back to the starting position. Pause for one second, then repeat.

PAY ATTENTION
Push from the shoulders as you extend your arms for maximum effect. Plus, make sure your lower back is pushed into the floor all the time throughout this exercise.

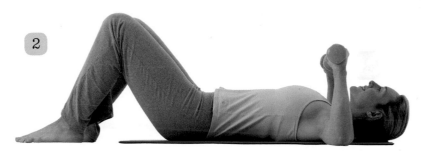

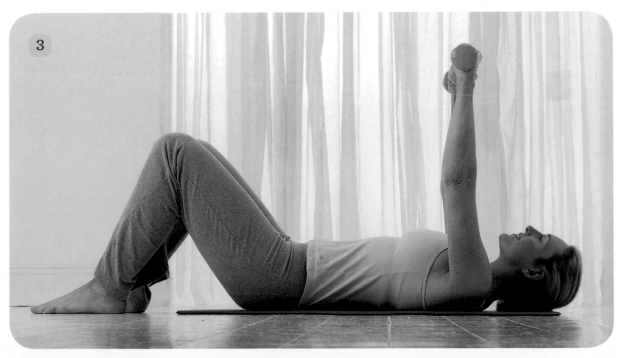

cooling-down exercises

Just as you need to warm up the body for exercising, you also need to cool it down after you have finished. Choose a few of the exercises shown over the next six pages, and take the time to cool down. Ideally, you should look to spend around ten minutes doing this.

post-exercise chest stretch

This stretch will help encourage deep breathing, which will enable you to feel a whole lot perkier and more refreshed in the morning.

1 Sit comfortably on the mat, cross-legged and with good posture. Lift your arms out to the sides and place them behind you.

2 Keep the shoulders down as you clasp your hands together.

3 Hold this stretch for 20 seconds.

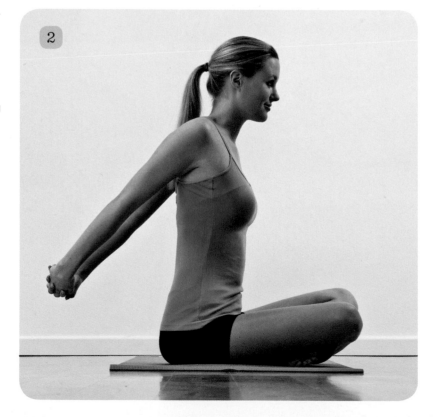

pec stretch

Your pectoral muscles (pecs) are the big muscles that sit under your bust. Stretching them out will help get rid of any knots or tension that may have built up from carrying heavy bags.

1 Stand with feet hips' width apart. Place your palms on your lower back, then gently pull your shoulders back together and stick your chest out until you feel the stretch. Keep your elbows soft.

2 Hold the stretch for three sets of ten seconds.

PAY ATTENTION

When you bring your shoulders back, be careful not to arch your back. All the movement should come from the shoulders.

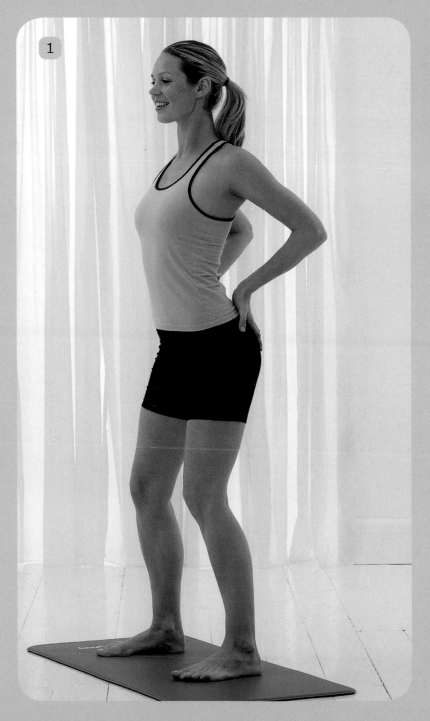

1

waist and lower spine

This is another great way of targeting your lower back muscles and really stretching them out. If you do it slowly and gently, it can even be good at soothing lower back problems.

1 Lie on the floor on your back with your legs straight out and your right arm extended out to the side.

2 Bending your right leg, grip your knee with your left hand and bring it over to your left-hand side so it gets as close to the floor as is comfortable. Keep your right hand extended out to your right-hand side because this will help to increase the stretch in your waist and lower spine.

3 Hold the stretch for two sets of ten seconds with a brief pause between. Repeat on your right side.

> ### PAY ATTENTION
> When you are stretching to the left side, make sure you keep the right hip on the floor and vice versa. This will stop you from stretching too far over and putting a strain on your lower back.

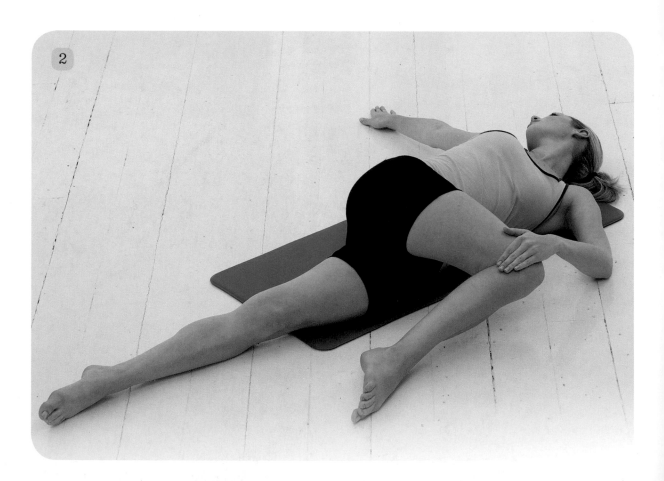

knee squeezes

The knee squeeze is a subtle way of stretching out the muscles across the middle of your back. This stretch feels very satisfying when done correctly, so spend some time making sure you get it right.

1 Lie on the floor with your knees bent and feet flat on the floor. Let your arms rest by your sides.

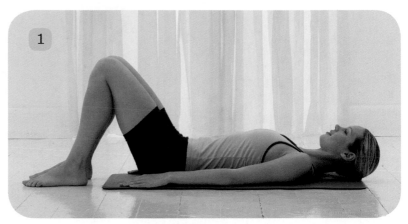

2 Gently bring your knees back toward your chest.

3 Engage your stomach muscles by pulling them in toward your spine and lift your tailbone ever so slightly off the floor. Grip your knees with your hands for support. You should feel a stretch across the middle of your back.

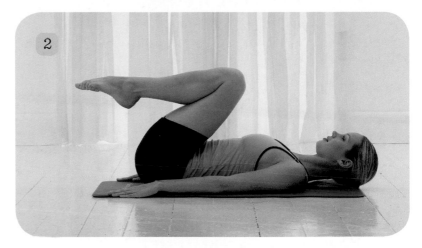

4 Hold the stretch for three sets of ten seconds, taking a very brief pause in between.

PAY ATTENTION

It's common to want to hold your breath during this stretch but make sure you don't. Breathe slowly and deeply and you will make the stretch easier to do and more effective.

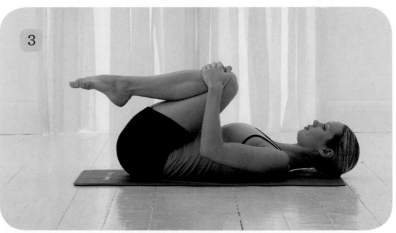

lower back stretch

This stretch is ideal for targeting the muscles across your lower back, which have a tendency to ache, especially if you've had a bad night's sleep. Stretching them in the morning will help to reduce your risk of injury during the day.

1 Stand with feet hips' width apart and knees slightly bent.

2 Place your hands on your inner thighs with your palms facing outward.

3 Engage your abdominals and slowly arch your spine until you feel a stretch across your lower back.

4 Hold for around ten seconds, then slowly stretch up through the spine until you are back in a normal standing position. Keep your back straight, with your chin up and looking forward.

5 Repeat the stretch three times.

PAY ATTENTION

If you're not feeling the stretch, simply move your palms farther down your thighs—this should help to increase it.

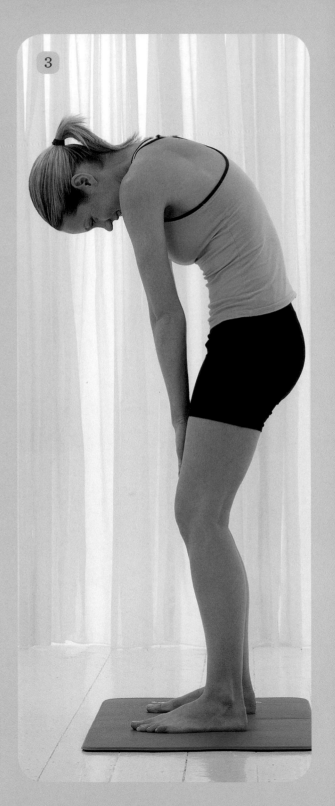

post-exercise upper back stretch

You will feel this stretch across your shoulders and the deep muscles of the back. Do not overstretch, because this should be a gentle movement.

1 Sit comfortably on the mat, cross-legged and with good posture. Lift up your arms in front of you.

2 Clasp your hands in front of you and imagine you are hugging a large ball. Feel the stretch in your back.

3 Hold this stretch for 20 seconds.

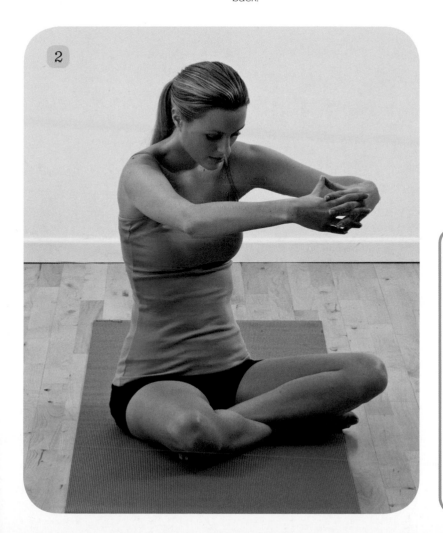

Train your brain

Use your mind to help you get the most from your workout. Focus on what you are doing correctly. As you are exercising tell yourself how well you are doing. Think of each muscle contracting and stretching as you do your routine. This can make you do even better, whereas concentrating on what you are doing wrong sets you up to fail. You can even use visualizations to convince yourself that your body is becoming fitter and more toned!

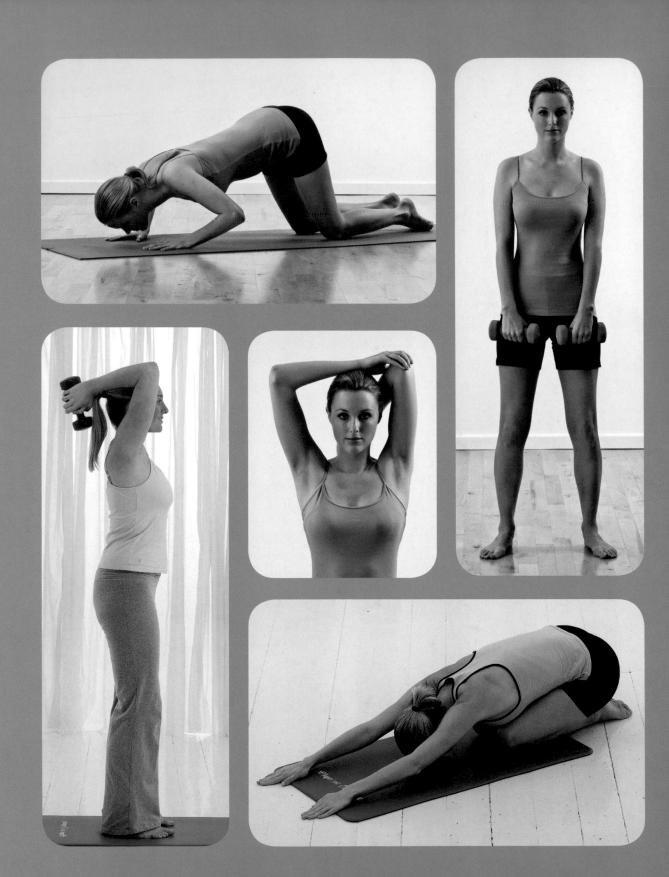

3

arms & shoulders

This chapter targets the key areas of your upper body. It will banish any wobble from your arms, tone your shoulders, and define and strengthen your back. Don't worry—these exercises won't bulk out your muscles, but will lengthen and define them, improve your posture, naturally lift your bust, and boost your confidence, too!

shrugs

This will help to release tension from the neck and shoulders.

1 Stand upright with your shoulder girdle and spine in neutral. Place your feet hips' width apart, keep your knees soft, and let your arms hang loosely by your sides. Focus on your breathing, with eyes closed if you want.

2 Inhale, and lift your shoulders up toward your ears.

3 Exhale, and draw the shoulder blades into neutral. At first, do the shrugs five times, increasing to a maximum of ten.

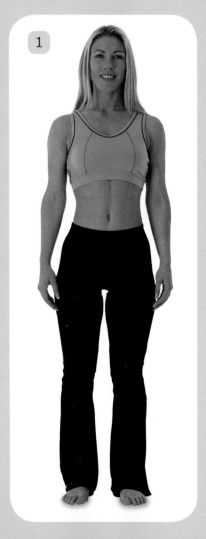

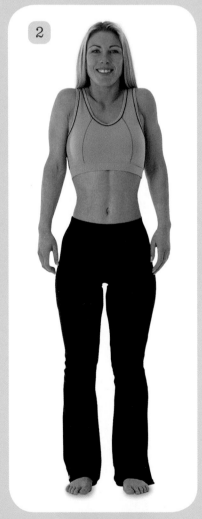

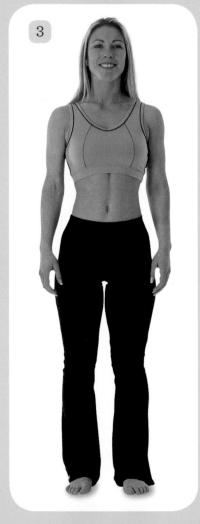

arm swing

This will increase the flexibility of your chest muscles and help to loosen your upper back.

1 Stand with good posture, knees bent and stomach pulled in.

2 Lift both arms out to either side of your body.

3 In a slow and controlled manner, bring both arms in front so they cross over, then back out to either side.

4 Be sure to keep your abdominal muscles pulled in to maintain good posture throughout.

5 Repeat the exercise ten times.

Mind over matter

Get the most from your workout by focusing on what you are doing as you are exercising, and tell yourself how well you are doing. You can even use visualizations as you exercise to convince yourself that your body is becoming fitter and more toned!

introductory exercises

These first-stage exercises are aimed at beginners, so you should find them relatively easy to start with, allowing you to become more involved as you progress. If you find any of the exercises a bit too difficult, feel free to replace them with something else of the same level.

sitting back toner

This trains the upper part of your arms, through your deltoid muscle.

1 Sit with good posture, feet hips' width apart and stomach pulled in.

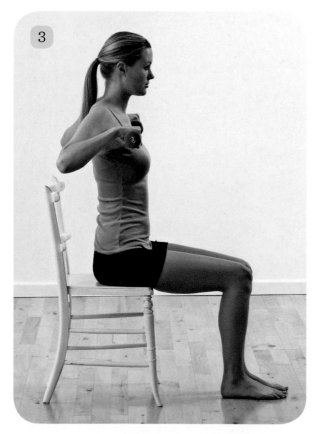

2 Holding a weight in each hand, lift your elbows up to shoulder height, then bend them so that your wrists are by your chest and your elbows are in line with your shoulders.

3 Using your weights, slowly squeeze both elbows behind you, maintaining the bend and keeping your elbows parallel to the floor. Hold for a second, then slowly return to the start position.

PAY ATTENTION

Aim to squeeze your shoulder blades together as you move your arms behind you.

Controlling your movements

Make sure that all exercises are performed slowly, carefully, and with your full attention. You really do need to concentrate on what you're doing and think about how your body is responding to any exercise.

If an action hurts or you do it too quickly, then you're not doing it properly. Movements should flow in a gentle, controlled manner. This enables your muscles to stretch naturally.

biceps curl

The biceps are the muscles at the front of the upper arms. They are relatively easy to tone, so practicing this exercise will help give you shapely arms that you'll want to show off.

1 Stand up tall with feet hips' width apart and knees soft.

2 Extend your arms out in front of you with palms facing upward, holding a dumbbell or a can of soup in each hand.

3 Bend your elbows and bring both your hands in toward your shoulders so that your arms form right-angles.

4 Reverse the movement so that your elbows are fully extended in front of you again. Keep your elbows soft at all times.

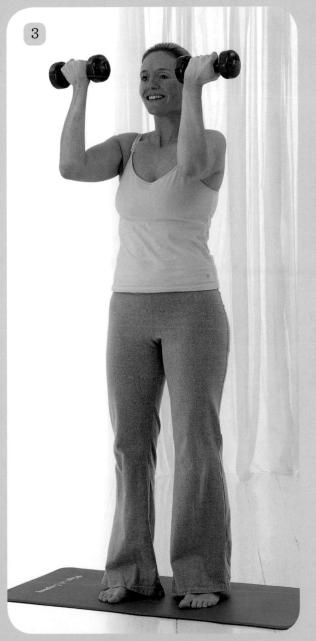

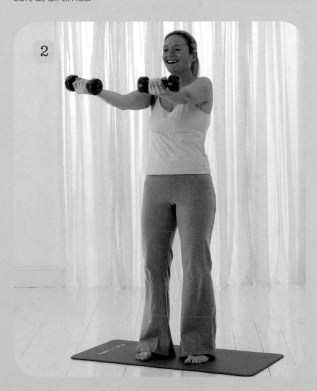

triceps squeeze back

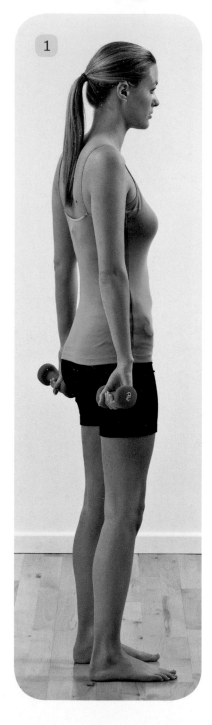

This is an easy-to-perform standing exercise that will tone through the back of your upper arms creating a long, toned triceps muscle and banishing any wobbly arms. The other great thing with this exercise is that it also stretches your chest muscles, which helps promote good posture.

1 Stand with good posture and your knees slightly bent. Hold the weights, keeping your arms by your side, with your palms facing away from you backward.

2 Lift your chest and pull your shoulders back.

3 Lift both arms directly behind you, and feel this working through your triceps. Hold your arms at the highest point, then slowly lower back to the start position.

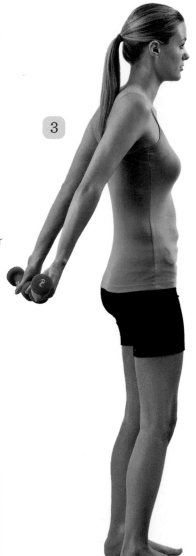

PAY ATTENTION

This is a small lift, so don't expect to raise your arms too high. Keep your knees slightly bent and your abdominal muscles pulled in tight.

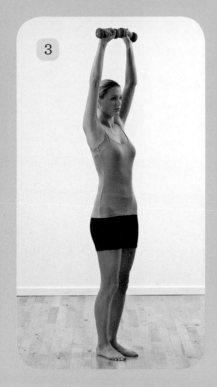

turning press

This is a great time-saving exercise, because it targets several upper body muscles at once, including your triceps, biceps, and shoulders.

1 Stand with your feet hips' width apart, upper body straight, knees soft, and stomach pulled in.

2 Hold a weight in each hand with the palms facing directly in front of your shoulders and your elbows bent as if in a biceps curl (see page 86).

3 Straighten elbows and lift weights overhead, twisting the hands until the palms face out. Lower your arms and twist your palms to face in again.

front raises

This exercise will sculpt your shoulders and create tone and definition through the front of your arms.

1 Stand with good posture, your feet hips' width apart and knees soft.

2 Keep your abdominal muscles tight and chest relaxed.

3 Hold a weight in each hand with palms facing in, weights by your thighs.

4 In a slow and controlled smooth move, lift both arms up forward and straight to shoulder height, then slowly lower both arms back to the start position.

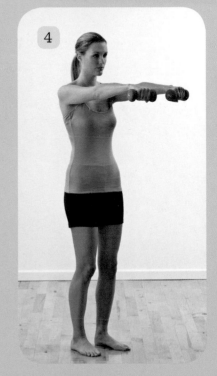

front arm toner (hammer curl)

This tones through the front of your upper arms and also works on strengthening your forearm muscles.

1 Stand with your feet shoulders' width apart, knees soft, elbows fixed, and stomach pulled in tight to promote good upper body posture.

2 With a weight in each hand, let both arms hang down long by the side of your body, fully straightened with your palms facing in toward your body.

3 Simultaneously lift your weights upward, without moving your elbows, hold for a second, then slowly lower back to your start position.

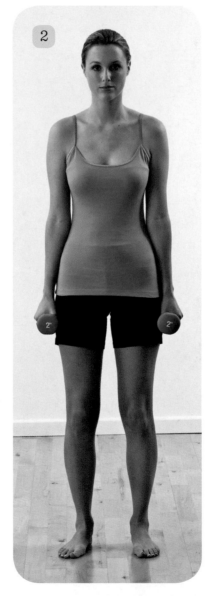

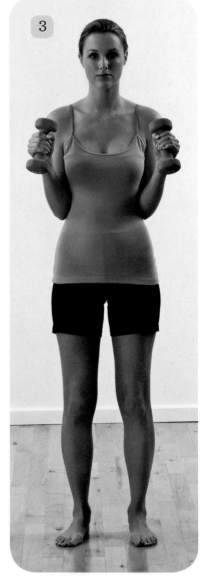

superwoman arms

This will tone through your shoulders and biceps, while working to improve your shoulder joint flexibility.

1 Kneel on the mat on all fours, with your wrists directly under your shoulders and your knees under your hips on the mat. Keep your abdominal muscles contracted. Holding a small weight, lift up one arm so that it is in line with your shoulder.

2 Now slowly bend the arm back so your elbow is then in line with your shoulder. Hold, then gently release back to a straight arm and repeat. Do all your repetitions on one arm and then repeat on the other arm.

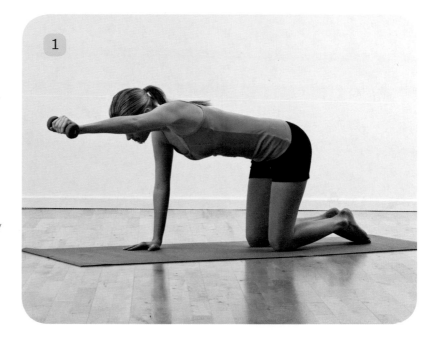

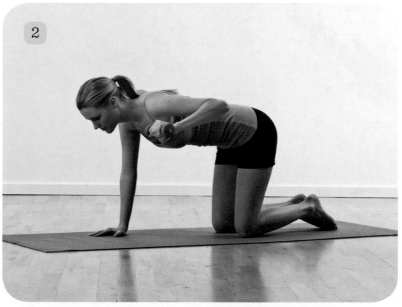

triceps extension

The triceps are the muscles at the back of the upper arms. If they're left to slack, it can lead to the dreaded flabby upper arm effect, where loose skin on the underside of your arm wobbles as you wave. It's classically a hard muscle to target, but this exercise will help to tighten and tone.

1 Stand with feet hips' width apart. Pick up a heavy object with both hands—choose something that you can work comfortably with, such as a dumbbell or a heavy book

2 Bring the object over your head with straight arms.

3 Bend your arms at the elbows, so you slowly lower it down between your shoulder blades.

4 Reverse the movement by straightening your arms so you bring the object directly back above your head.

5 Repeat Steps 3 and 4 slowly, so you're in control of the movement.

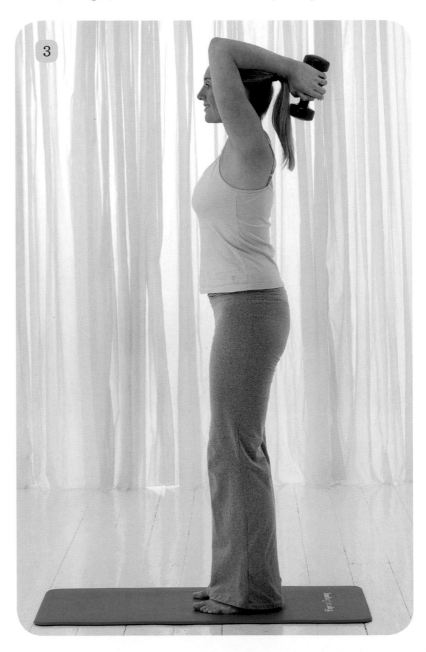

PAY ATTENTION

Choose a weight that's challenging but not so heavy that you can't control it—you don't want to end up dropping it on your head.

kneeling box push-up

This exercise targets a lot of your upper body and arm muscles so it is great for toning your arms, your bust, and also for building upper body strength. You will notice the fitter and the more toned your arms become, the stronger you will be, and you should soon be able to perform these with ease.

1 Kneel on the mat with knees directly under your hips. Hands should be slightly wider than shoulders' width apart, with fingers pointing forward.

2 Keep your body weight over your hands, stomach pulled in tight, and your back flat. Slowly lower your body so your elbows are at a 90-degree angle.

3 Gently push yourself back up to the start position.

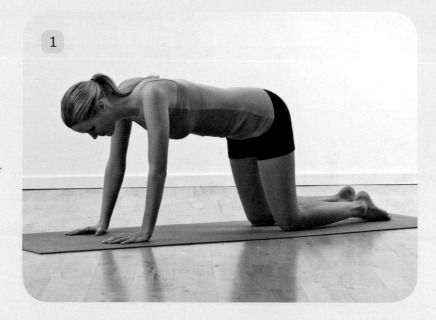

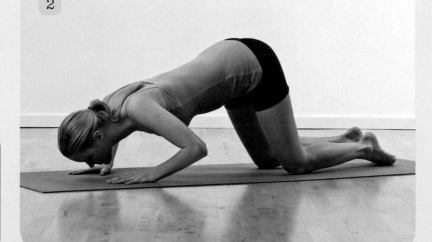

Lifting weights

When lifting weights, always keep the movement slow and controlled. This not only works the muscles harder but it also prevents any injuries occurring.

side shoulder raise

This exercise will help to define your shoulders—it is also good for improving flexibility throughout your shoulder joints and will give you good posture.

1 Stand with your feet shoulders' width apart and your knees slightly bent.

2 Hold the hand weights at your sides at thigh level.

3 Slowly lift the weights out to the sides to shoulder level, keeping your elbows slightly bent. Keep your shoulders down and relaxed as you lift. If you find you are shrugging your shoulders up toward your ears, your weights may be too heavy.

4 Slowly lower the weights back to your start position.

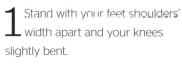

PAY ATTENTION

It's important to keep a slight bend in both arms as you lift them. Imagine both arms are pouring a cup of coffee, because, as this helps to keep the arms soft.

triceps ponytail

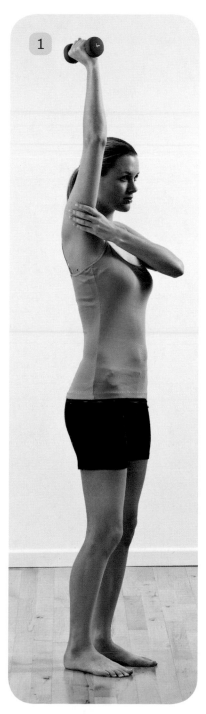

This standing triceps exercise is one of the best ways to tone flabby upper arms.

1 Stand with good posture. Bend your knees slightly and pull in your stomach. Place a weight in your right hand, then extend the right arm straight up and support it with the other arm. Keep a good posture and your abdominal muscles pulled in.

2 Now simply bend at the elbow of your extended arm so the weight is by your upper back. Slowly straighten the arm back up to the start position. Do all your repetitions on one arm and then repeat on the other arm.

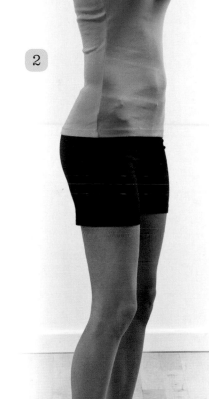

PAY ATTENTION
The arm that supports your exercising arm keeps the elbow in line with your shoulder.

arm opener

This exercise works by toning the biceps in your front upper arms. The exercise will firm the biceps, not bulk them out.

1 Stand with your feet shoulders' width apart, knees soft, elbows fixed, and stomach pulled in tight to promote good upper body posture.

2 Have your arms by your side with your elbows bent and your arms in an L shape, a weight in each hand.

3 With your palms facing in toward each other, slowly open your forearms out to either side, while still keeping your elbows tucked into your sides. Hold for a second, then slowly return to a start position.

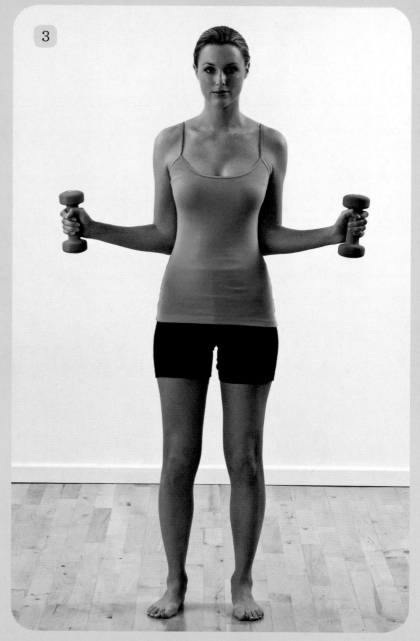

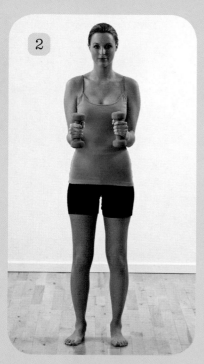

upright pull

This exercise focuses on toning through your shoulders, biceps, and back, which will help you achieve a beautifully toned upper body.

1 Stand with your feet shoulders' width apart and your knees slightly bent.

2 Hold a weight in each hand, side by side at thigh level, keeping your palms facing toward your thighs.

3 Slowly bring the weights up toward your collarbone, until your elbows are about shoulder height. Keep your shoulders down and relaxed as you lift. If you find you are shrugging your shoulders up toward your ears, your weights may be too heavy.

4 Slowly lower the weights to the start position.

> **PAY ATTENTION**
> Ensure you keep your weights close to your body as you lift and lower them.

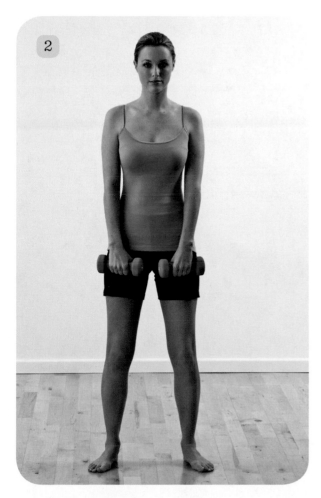

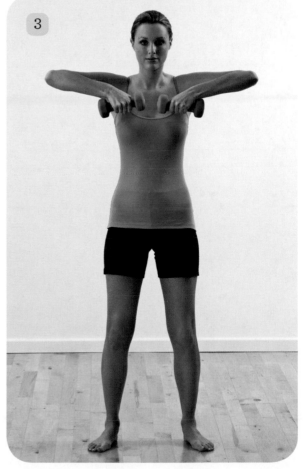

triceps dips

This exercise specifically works on toning your triceps by working both arms in one move. You will notice how quickly this muscle tones up and that this exercise will feel easier each week as the arms become fitter.

1 Sit right on the edge of your chair, with your hands next to your hips and your palms face down.

2 Place your feet firmly on the floor hips' width apart and with your knees bent.

3 Lift up onto your hands and bring your hips slightly forward.

4 Bend your elbows and lower your hips down, keeping them very close to the chair. Keep your abdominal muscles pulled in and shoulders down.

5 In a controlled manner, slowly push back up without locking the elbows.

PAY ATTENTION
Make sure you keep your hips close to the chair to keep the focus on your triceps and not on your shoulders.

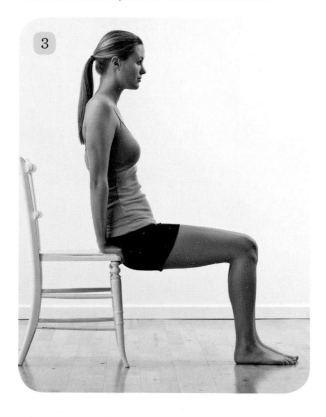

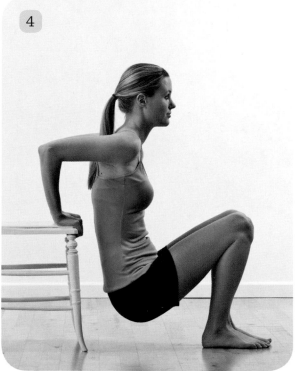

floor arm lift

This is a challenging exercise but it is fantastic for sculpting your upper arms because it really works your triceps.

1 Sit on the mat with your legs straight and together. Place your hands, fingertips forward, just behind your hips, and point your toes.

2 Pull in your abdominal muscles, straighten your arms (hands should be under your shoulders), and lift your hips off the floor until your body is aligned from shoulders to toes. Keep looking forward.

3 Hold the position for a second, then slowly lower.

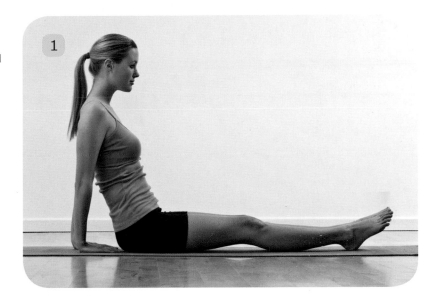

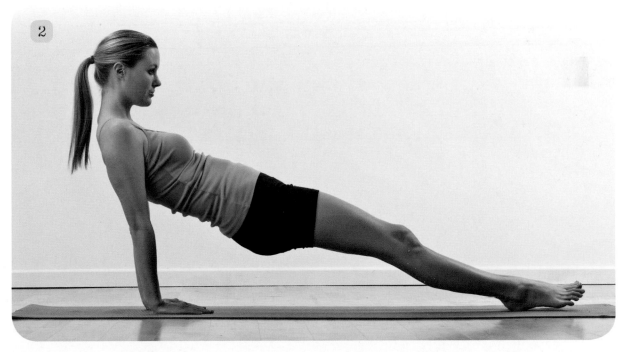

cooling-down exercises

Just as you need to warm up the body for exercising, you also need to cool it down after you have finished. Choose a few of the exercises shown over the next six pages, and take the time to cool down. Ideally, you should look to spend around ten minutes doing this.

triceps stretch

Your triceps muscles are found at the back of the top of your arms. Giving them a good stretch will boost circulation and help to get rid of any blotchy, pimply skin that may reside there.

1 Stand with good posture, lift one arm above your head and drop the palm of the hand behind the head between the shoulder blades.

2 Lift the other arm and support the stretching arm on the soft, fleshy part of the upper arm or just above the elbow.

3 Hold this stretch for 15 seconds. Repeat on the other arm.

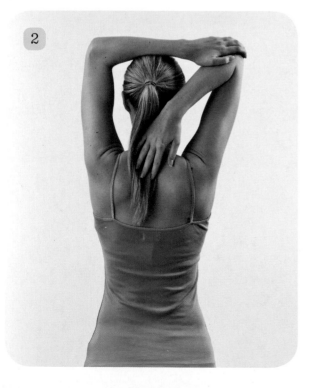

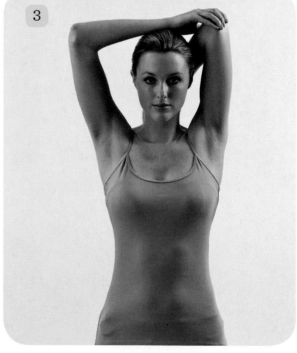

seashell stretch

This stretch is great at targeting the muscles in your shoulders as well as your back. Just sit back and relax and you will feel the beneficial effects of the stretch.

1 Get down on the floor on your hands and knees. Sit back on your calves, so your backside is resting on your heels. Make sure your neck and head are relaxed and that you are looking down toward the floor.

2 Stretch your arms out in front of you so that your hands and fingertips are spread on the floor.

3 Walk your hands as far forward as you can until you can feel the stretch in the middle of your back.

4 Hold the stretch for three sets of ten seconds.

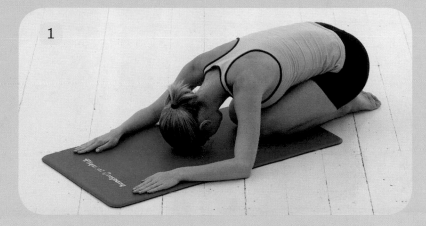

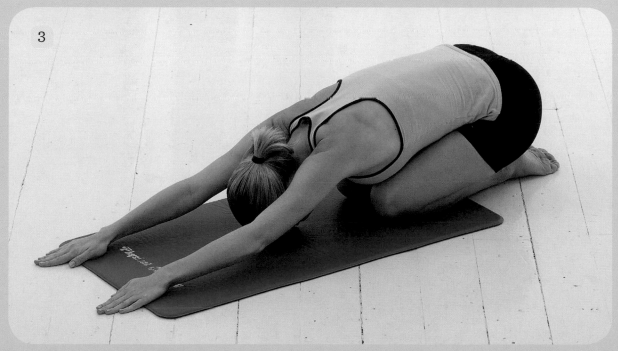

chest stretch

If you spend a lot of time using a computer, your shoulders tend to draw in and rise upward. The chest stretch is good for counteracting this movement and helps to open up the shoulder and chest area.

1 Stand with good posture with your feet slightly apart.

2 Clasp your hands together behind your back, and raise them until you feel the stretch in your chest.

3 Keep your shoulders down as you hold onto your wrists.

4 Hold this position for ten seconds.

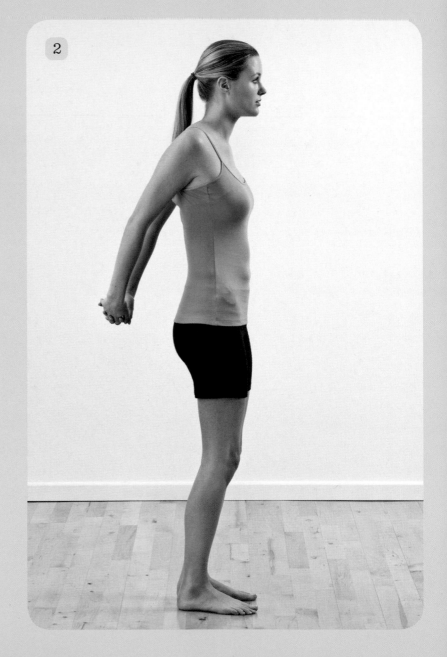

shoulder stretch

This is an easy stretch to do, and will really get your shoulders loosened up. It's great to do if you've been particularly stressed out recently, because it will help to get rid of any built-up tension.

1 You can do this stretch from either a standing or a sitting position. Extend your right arm directly out in front of you so it's parallel with the floor.

2 Using your left hand, grip the back of your right arm between your elbow and your shoulder and use it to bring your right arm gently across the front of your chest. You should feel the stretch down the inner side of your right arm and across your right shoulder blade.

3 Hold the position for two sets of ten seconds and then repeat with the other arm.

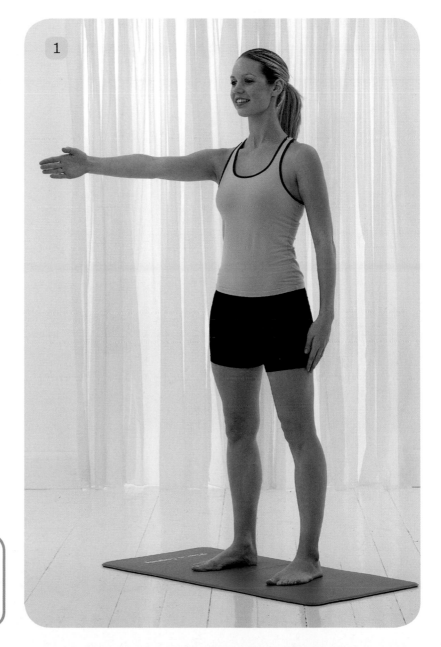

PAY ATTENTION

Stop yourself from rotating by making sure your hips are facing forward at all times.

inner arm stretch

This targets all the muscles in your upper arms—you'll be surprised at how easy it is to feel the stretch.

1 Stand in an open door frame, with your abs tight and body straight.

2 Hold onto the doorjamb with your left hand just below shoulder level, or as high as is comfortable. Take a big step forward so your left arm is extended out behind you. Keeping your hips facing forward and your head and neck in line with your spine, rotate your upper body to the right until you feel the stretch in your left arm. Lean forward to feel a greater stretch.

3 Hold for two sets of ten seconds, then turn around, step forward, and repeat the stretch with your right arm.

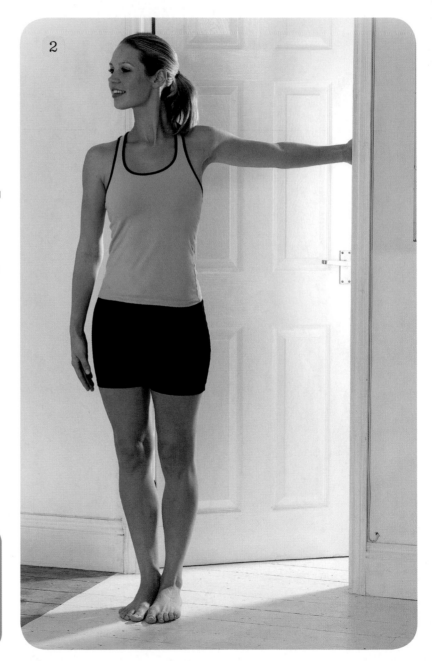

PAY ATTENTION

Don't worry if you find it difficult to get your arm up to shoulder height because you can still achieve a good stretch by having it slightly lower.

biceps stretch

The bicep muscles are the big muscles at the front of your upper arms. It's good to stretch them out so you develop long, lean arms that look great in sleeveless tops!

1 Stand with feet hips' width apart, stomach muscles pulled in, and hands resting by your sides.

2 Extend your right arm out in front of you with your palm flat, facing the floor.

3 Extend your left arm, placing the left palm under the right palm. Gently push your hands against each other. You will feel the stretch in your biceps.

4 Hold for three sets of ten seconds, then repeat for the other arm.

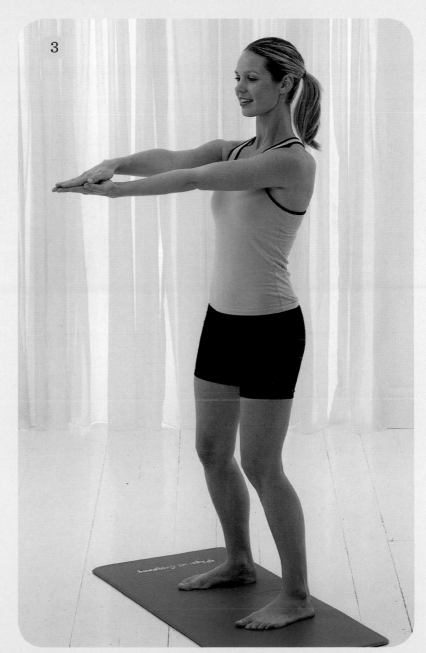

PAY ATTENTION

Don't try to force your hands together with a lot of pressure. Just take it slowly and start with a small amount of pressure in order to achieve a gentle stretch.

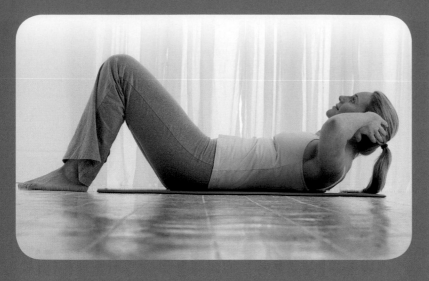

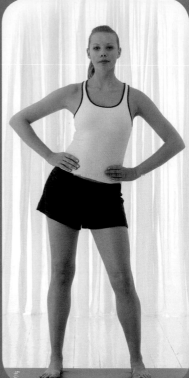

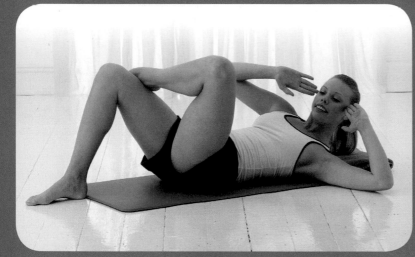

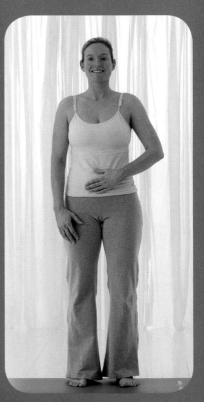

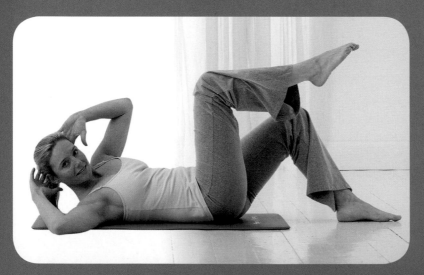

4

stomach

Most of us would love to have a flatter stomach but just can't face the thought of hours and hours of strenuous sit-ups. Well, the good news is you don't have to do this—the key to a fit and toned stomach is to exercise little and often. Just follow the routines in this section and you'll have a flatter stomach within weeks.

introduction

As well as looking fantastic, a flat stomach increases your flexibility, improves posture, and helps keep the body in good working order. Strengthening the stomach muscles can even help lower the risk of heart disease, high blood pressure, and diabetes.

The benefits

Apart from the obvious benefit of improving your appearance, firming and toning up your stomach muscles will improve your posture and balance, and increase your flexibility. Building muscle tone doesn't happen overnight, but the varied range of exercises in this section means that you won't become bored or burned out. Keep it up and you'll have a tighter stomach in no time.

Stomach muscles explained

It helps to have a basic understanding of which muscles you need to work on to make your stomach appear flatter.

There are four abdominal muscle groups, which form a natural corset around the middle. They support your lower back, protect internal organs, and enable you to

bend, twist, and sit up. The deepest of the abdominal muscles is the transversus abdominis, which wraps horizontally around your waist and keeps your lower back stable. The rectus abdominis runs from the pubic bone to the bottom of the rib cage. This muscle enables your trunk to bend and is important for maintaining your posture.

The external and internal obliques run up the sides of your body and enable you to bend to the side and twist your spine. The exercises in this section will work to strengthen all these muscles for a firmer, flatter, fabulously toned stomach.

Effective exercising

When you start out, make sure you don't overdo it; just do as many reps as you can comfortably achieve. To make it effective, it's important that you don't stop for more than

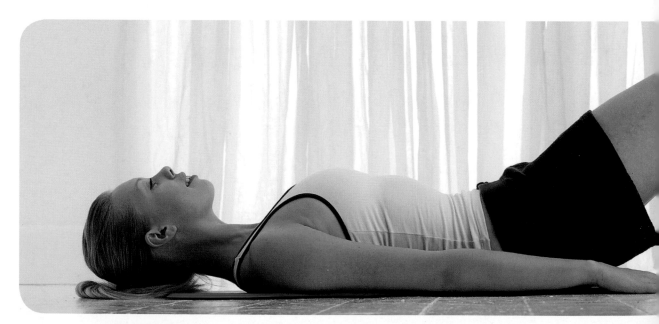

a minute between exercises. Shorter recovery periods result in better muscles all round and improved muscle endurance. So keep going!

Handy hints for a flabby stomach

Learning how to pull your abdominal muscles in can help strengthen them.

• With the stomach muscles relaxed, measure and cut a length of ribbon or string to fit the waist and tie it around.

• As you breathe out, pull the navel in. The objective is to keep any tension off the string by maintaining this hold. Take five breaths, then exhale. Repeat eight times.

Practice makes perfect and this isn't easy, but when you have achieved holding your stomach in flat without relying on the string it will come as second nature, even when exercising, and ultimately this will ensure you get the best from every workout.

What you'll need

For this section, you'll need a sturdy chair, a nonslip mat, a cushion, and a pillow or towel to support your head and neck. Don't forget to warm up and cool down!

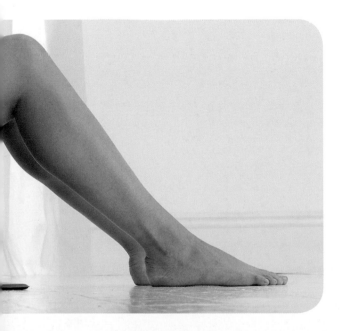

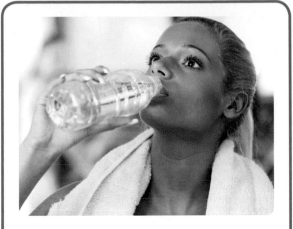

Eating for a flat stomach

Adopting a few healthy eating tips can help beat bloating and boost the effects of exercise.

Don't ever skimp on liquids if you think it could ward off bloating because drinking a lot of water actually promotes a flat stomach by flushing toxins from your system and curbing your appetite. If your body feels starved of water, then it will hold onto what there is, which can lead to water retention and the appearance of bloating.

Drink at least eight glasses a day, but don't drink a lot before exercise because it will put pressure on your bladder. You'll know you're well hydrated by checking the color of your urine—the paler it is, the better.

If your stomach has a noticeable wobble, you will have to do some regular cardiovascular exercise to promote fat loss and these healthy eating tips will also help:

• Eat little and often and make sure you have a varied diet. Keep wheat products to a minimum because they can cause bloating and gas in people sensitive to wheat or gluten.

• Say good-bye to carbonated drinks—even if they're "diet" or caffeine-free, they can still cause bloating because they are loaded with gassy bubbles.

• Avoid processed food and prepared meals. They are usually laden with salt, sugar, and chemicals, and can upset your stomach's bacterial balance and cause bloating.

• Cut down on salt—it can encourage fluid retention.

warming-up exercises

It is always essential to warm up before undertaking any form of exercise. Choose a couple of the exercises shown over the next few pages and spend a little time warming up. You should allow around ten minutes for this, and alternate them so you don't get bored.

waist twist

It's important not to move your hips and knees during this exercise, but do feel free to move your arms like a hula dancer if it helps you get into the right mood!

1 Stand up straight with your spine in neutral and your knees slightly bent (soft, not "locked"). Keep your feet hips' width apart and your hands resting on your hips. Make sure your spine is in the neutral position.

2 Tighten your abdominal muscles by pulling your navel back toward your spine.

3 Keeping your hips and knees still, rotate your shoulders and head to the right, then return to the center.

4 Now twist to the left, rotating your head and shoulders and keeping your hips and knees still.

5 Repeat this exercise another five times on each side.

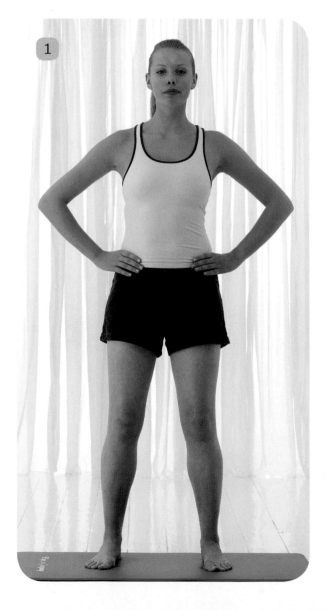

1

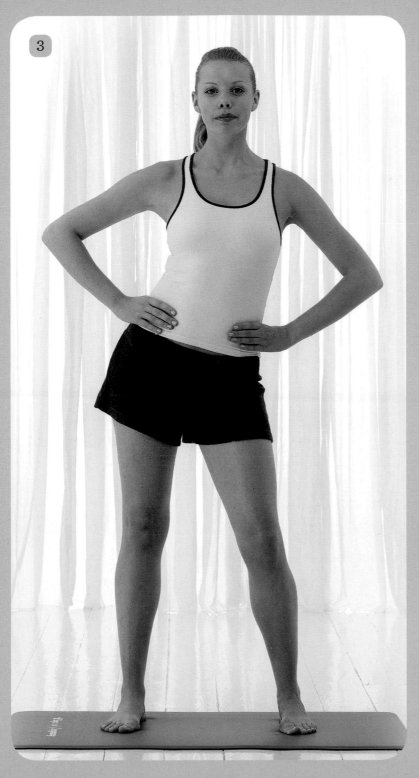

3

hip circles

This exercise will mobilize your lower abdominal muscles. Try to make sure that only your pelvis is rocking instead of moving your torso.

1 Stand up straight with your knees slightly bent, feet hips' width apart, hands resting on your hips.

2 Tighten your abdominal muscles by gently pulling your navel toward your spine. This movement should feel light and subtle—do not suck in your waist or hold your breath.

3 Gently rotate your pelvis to the right so that you are rotating in a full circle.

4 Repeat nine times to the right, then circle ten times to the left.

forward bend

With this exercise, bend only as far as is comfortable—you don't have to touch your toes. Remember, you'll be able to stretch farther as time goes by and you become more supple with exercise.

1 Stand up straight with your feet hips' width apart and your knees slightly bent, not locked. Place your hands palms downward on the front of your thighs.

2 Tighten your abdominal muscles by gently pulling in your navel toward your backbone.

3 Slowly slide your hands down your legs toward your toes. Try not to overarch your back.

4 Position yourself so you feel a stretch in the hamstrings at the back of your legs but don't stretch so far that it hurts.

5 Hold for a count of three, then return to the center.

6 Repeat five more times. Keep your breathing steady throughout.

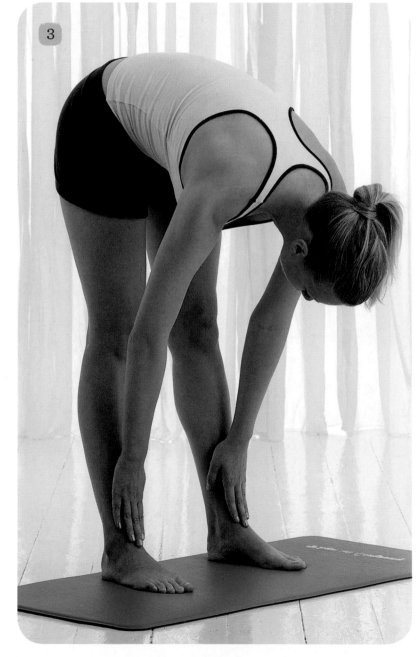

side bends

Do not do this exercise quickly with your arms above your head because this will make it hard to control the movement.

1 Stand up straight with your feet hips' width apart and your knees slightly bent, your arms by your sides.

2 Tighten your abdominal muscles by gently pulling your navel toward your spine.

3 Keeping your back straight and without leaning forward, slowly bend to one side from the waist so that your hand slides down the side of your leg. Straighten up again.

4 Repeat on the other side. Repeat five more times on both sides.

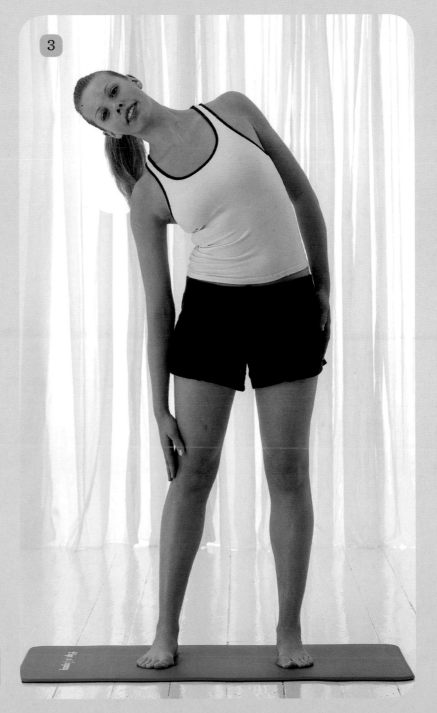

> **PAY ATTENTION**
> Never stretch to the point of pain.

stomach tuck-in

This exercise is like the natural alternative to wearing a corset. It works the deep muscles in your stomach—the transverse abdominals—to help flatten and define the muscles. It's the perfect start to getting a superflat stomach.

1 Stand with feet hips' width apart and hands resting by your sides.

2 Slowly contract your abdominals (your stomach muscles) by pulling them in toward your spine, but don't hold your breath. If you put your hand to your stomach, you should feel the muscles tighten—this means they're working. For best results, really concentrate on what you're doing and how it feels.

3 Slowly release and get ready to start again.

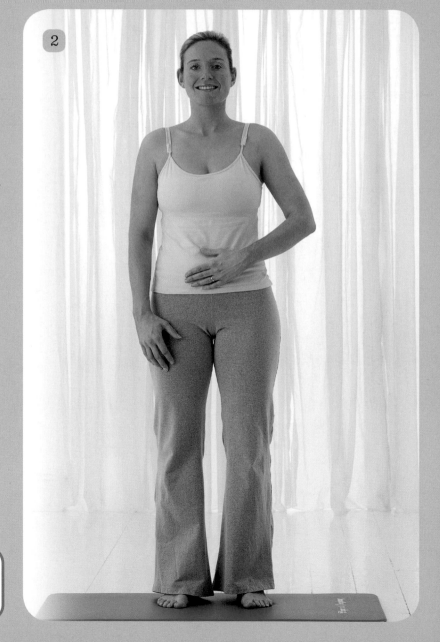

PAY ATTENTION
This exercise can also be done sitting on a chair.

up and over

This exercise is an old-style way of targeting the muscles at the side of your waist, which are called the "obliques". It's a great way of stretching out your love handles and it also helps you to feel really refreshed in the morning.

1 Stand with feet hips' width apart and your hands resting by your sides. Make sure your legs are slightly bent with knees soft. Keep your back straight and your head and neck in line with your spine.

2 Raise your left arm over your head and lean over from the waist to the right, so that your right hand travels down the side of your right leg. Your left arm should be reaching up and over your head. You should feel the stretch in the left side of your waist.

3 Hold for two sets of ten seconds, then slowly return to the starting position and repeat on the other side.

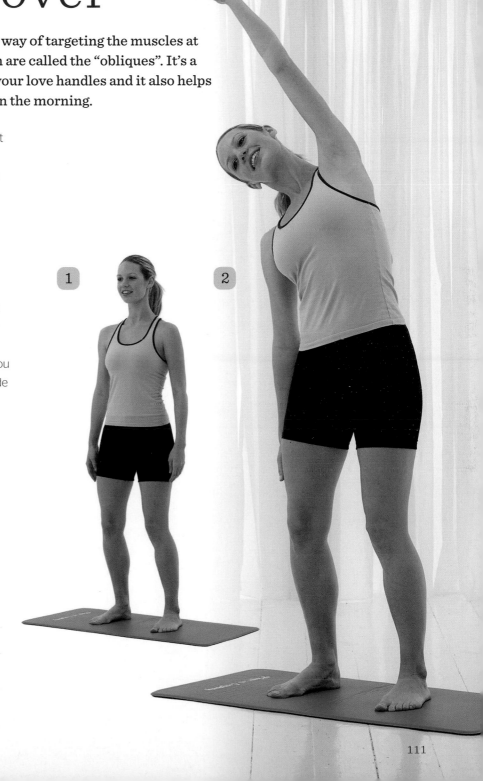

introductory exercises

These first-stage exercises are aimed at beginners, so you should find them relatively easy to start with, allowing you to become more involved as you progress. If you find any of the exercises a bit too difficult, feel free to replace them with something else of the same level.

belly tightener

This is also known as abdominal hollowing and helps to shorten the abdominal muscles, which is good for your posture and creates the appearance of a flatter stomach.

1 Kneel down on all fours (the "box" position) with your hands shoulders' width apart, your elbows slightly bent and your knees under your hips. Keep your head in line with the rest of your body and look down at the floor, making sure that your chin isn't tucked into your chest.

2 Relax your abdominal muscles, then slowly draw in your navel toward your spine.

3 Hold the muscles in for a count of ten, then slowly relax. Breathe slowly and steadily throughout this exercise.

> **PAY ATTENTION**
> Pull up the abdomen by using your deep abdominal muscles, not by arching your spine.

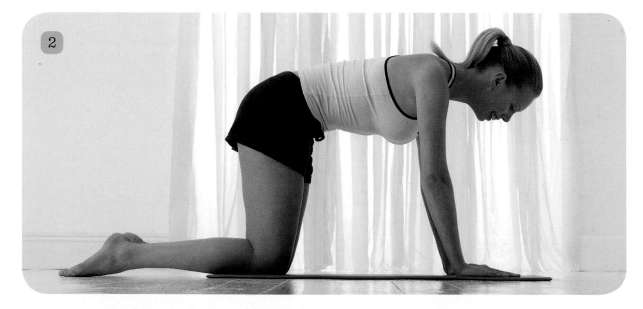

side reach

The small, controlled movements in this exercise work your stomach muscles even harder.

1 Lie on your back with your spine in neutral, your knees bent, feet flat on the floor, hips' width apart, and palms down and by your sides. Tighten your abdominal muscles.

2 Lift your head and shoulders off the floor to an angle of 30 degrees. Hold this position and reach out with your right hand toward your right calf.

3 Gently move back and forth ten times, then curl back down again. Remember to breathe regularly throughout.

4 Now repeat this exercise, reaching out with the left hand toward the left calf. Gradually build up the number of reaches you can do.

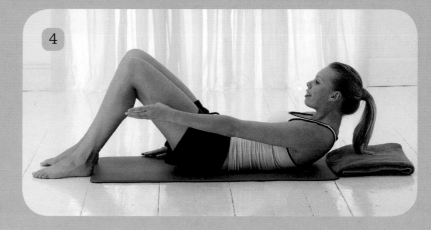

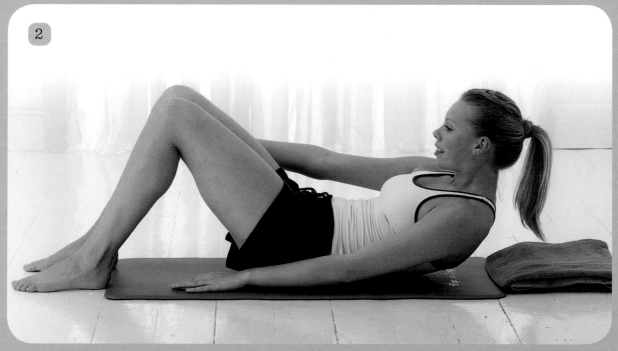

sitting knee lift

This sitting exercise will work your rectus abdominis—the muscle that runs down the front of your stomach. Make sure your movements are controlled and flowing.

1 Sit on the edge of a chair with your knees bent and pressed together and your feet flat on the floor. Hold onto the sides of the chair, then tighten your stomach muscles.

2 Lean back slightly and lift your feet just a little off the ground, keeping your knees bent and pressed together.

3 Slowly pull your knees in toward your chest and curl your upper body forward. Then lower your feet to the floor. Rest for a count of three before you do any repetitions.

> **PAY ATTENTION**
> Don't lean too far forward or you'll fall off the chair!

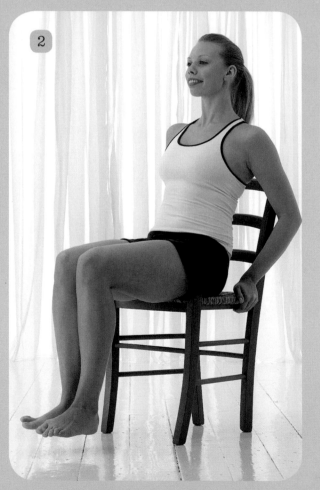

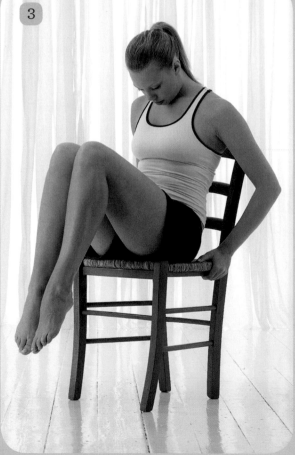

spine rotation

This exercise gently mobilizes your spine, preparing it for harder exercises to come.

1 Sit forward on a chair with your back straight and your hands resting on your thighs. Your knees should be over your ankles.

2 Tighten your abdominal muscles. Keeping your hips and knees forward, slowly rotate your upper body to the left until you can put both hands on the back of the chair. Hold for a count of ten, then return to the center. Repeat the exercise, twisting to the right.

Don't exercise if...

- you are feeling unwell—your body will need all its strength to fight off any infection.
- you have an injury—you might make things worse.
- you have an ongoing medical condition or are on medication—consult your doctor first.
- you've just had a big meal.
- you've been drinking alcohol.

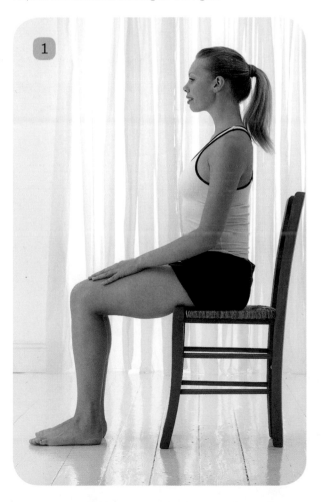

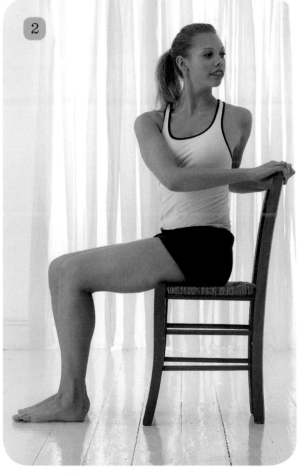

leg slide

Another easy exercise for tightening your stomach muscles.

1 Lie on your back with your knees bent, your feet flat on the floor, and your arms by your sides, palms facing the floor. You can put a flat pillow or towel under your neck for support, if you like.

2 Tighten your abdominal muscles by gently pulling in your navel toward your backbone.

3 Gently tilt your pelvis so that the pelvic bone rises.

4 Raising the toes of one foot, breathe out while sliding your leg forward as far as it will go, with your heel on the floor.

5 Hold for a count of three, then return to the starting position and repeat using the other leg.

How muscles work

Here's the science: Muscles are made up of millions of tiny protein filaments that relax and contract to produce movement. Most muscles are attached to bones by tendons and are consciously controlled by your brain. Electrical signals from the brain travel via nerves to the muscles, causing the cells within the muscle to contract. Movement happens when muscles pull on tendons, which move the bones at the joints. Muscles work in pairs, enabling bones to move in two directions, and most movements require the use of several muscle groups.

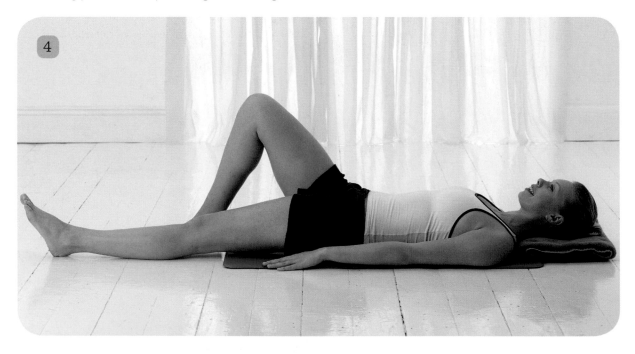

4

simple pelvic tilt

These exercises tighten the abdominal muscles without putting any strain on your back. They're a simple way to tone and strengthen your abdominal area.

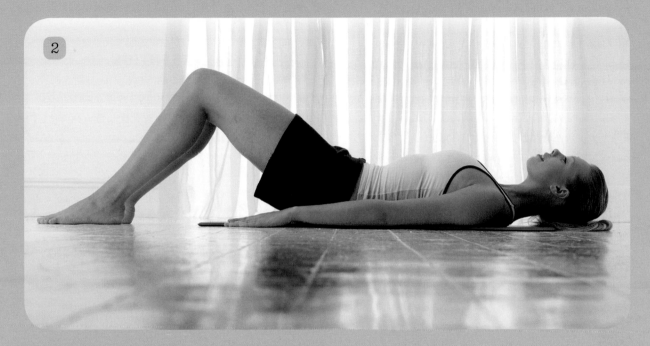

1 Lie on your back with your knees bent and feet flat on the floor, hips' width apart, and your spine in neutral. Rest your arms by your sides, palms facing the floor, and tighten your abdominal muscles.

2 Press your lower back down into the floor and gently tilt your pelvis so that the pubic bone rises, then tilt it back down.

3 Repeat several times, using a slow, steady rhythm.

Setting the pace

It's important to work at the right intensity if you're toning up—put in too little effort and you won't notice much difference; throw yourself into the exercises and you may hurt yourself. The aim of a toning program is to make your muscles work harder, either by increasing the time you exercise or by increasing the intensity of your workout. Your muscles will start to become tired during the last repetitions and you may feel a burning sensation in the area you're working, but this is normal and will pass as soon as you rest. Muscle soreness and stiffness is highly likely in the beginning, particularly if you're new to exercise, but if you can hardly move, then you've overdone it. Rest for a day or so and start again at a reduced intensity.

119

advanced exercises

Now that you've worked through the introductory exercises and are feeling more confident and fitter, you can progress to this second series of exercises. As before, if you find any particular exercises too difficult, feel free to replace them with something else from this level.

crunches

This is an intense workout for your stomach muscles and a great way of getting a washboard-flat stomach.

1 Lie on the floor, knees bent and feet apart, flat on the floor in line with your hips. Make sure your lower back is pressed into the floor. Put your hands behind your head to support your neck.

PAY ATTENTION
Make sure you don't use your neck to pull yourself up.

2 Engage your stomach muscles by pulling your abdominals toward your spine, and lift your upper body off the floor as far as you can without arching your lower back. You may find that you can't get up very high, but it's the effort of moving that counts, so make sure that you're pushing yourself as hard as you comfortably can. With practice, you may be able to sit up completely.

3 When you can't go any farther, pause for one second. Then gently lower yourself back down into the starting position.

PAY ATTENTION
Don't use your hands to lift your head off the floor—let your stomach muscles do all the work.

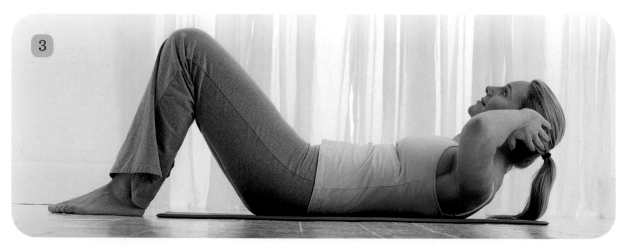

side lift

This exercise works the obliques and reinforces your body's natural alignment. Make sure you don't use the supporting arm to push yourself up—the movement is controlled by the stomach muscles.

1 Lie on your side in a straight line. Extend your lower arm above your head in line with your body. Bend your top arm in front to support you—your hand should be in line with your chest.

2 Tighten your abdominal muscles, then lift both legs together off the floor.

3 Now raise your upper leg higher, keeping it aligned with the bottom leg.

4 Hold for a count of two, then lower the top leg to the bottom leg.

5 Lower both legs slowly to the floor. Repeat on the other side of your body.

PAY ATTENTION

Both these exercises are great waist-whittlers but you may find them too hard if you're a beginner—you should be able to do these after a few weeks of stomach-toning exercise.

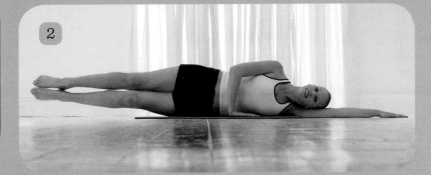

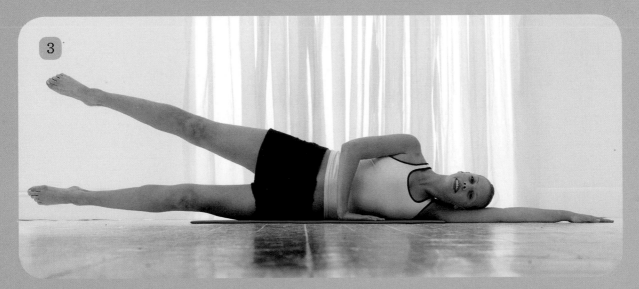

bicycle

This is similar to the crunches exercise, featured previously, but crossing your elbow to the opposite knee targets the obliques instead, which are found at the side of the waist. Practicing this exercise will help give you a smaller, more defined middle.

1 Lie on the floor with your knees bent and feet flat on the floor.

2 Rest your hands behind your head and, using your stomach muscles, lift your upper body off the floor, making sure that your lower back stays firmly on the floor.

3 Lift your right foot off the floor and bring your right knee toward your chest.

4 Reach forward and rotate from the waist slightly in order to bring your left elbow toward your right knee. They don't have to touch.

5 Pause for one second, then return to the starting position. Repeat the movement, bringing your right knee toward your left elbow.

6 Continue the exercise on alternate sides.

> ### PAY ATTENTION
> Make sure your head and neck are in line with your spine and that you're looking up toward the ceiling—it will prevent you from straining your neck.

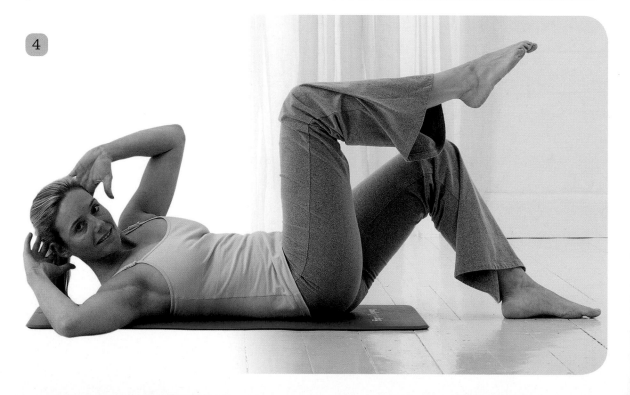

4

lower abdominal raise

This is a harder exercise that will really work your abdominal muscles. If it seems easy, then you're not doing it properly!

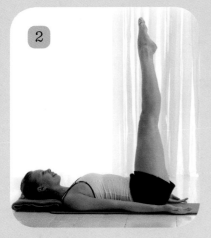

1 Lie on your back with your knees bent, feet flat on the floor and hips' width apart. Make sure your spine is in neutral. Keep your arms by your sides with the palms facing upward.

2 Lift your legs into the air, one at a time, until they reach an angle of 90 degrees to your body.

3 Tighten your abdominal muscles and slowly lower one foot to the floor, then bring it back up again. Repeat this exercise using the other leg.

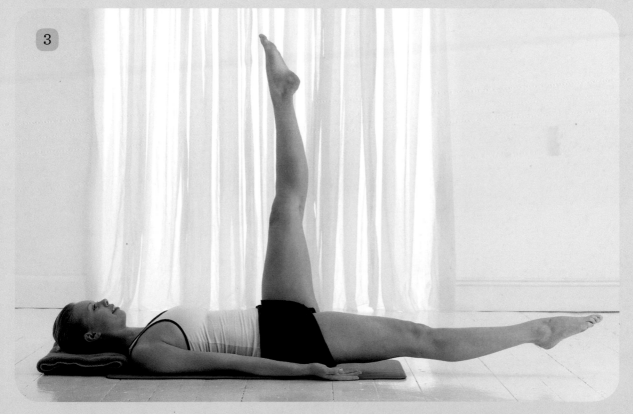

slightly harder reverse curl

Never do full sit-ups—curling is much safer and more effective.

1 Lie on your back with your spine in neutral. You can keep your hands by the sides of your head or rest your arms by your sides with the palms facing downward. Keep your legs up vertically with the knees bent and your ankles crossed over. Tighten your abdominal muscles.

2 Tilt your pelvis forward so that your backside lifts off the floor, keeping your legs still as you do so. Lower your pelvis to the start position.

Controlling your movements

Make sure that all exercises are performed slowly, carefully, and with your full attention. You really do need to concentrate on what you're doing and think about how your body is responding to any exercise. If an action hurts or you do it quickly, then you're not doing it properly. Movements should flow in a gentle, controlled manner.

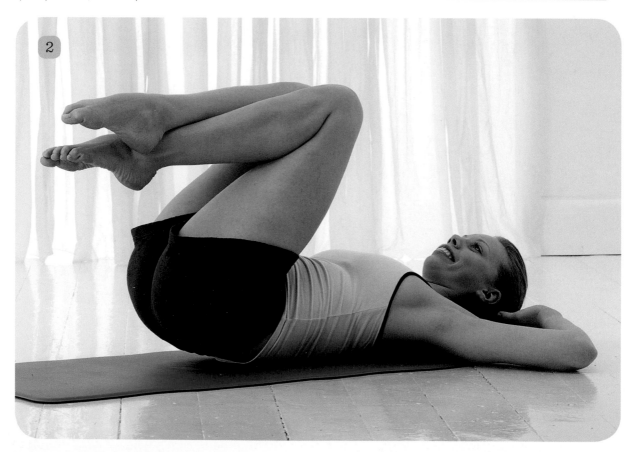

pillow roll

This exercise tones and strengthens your obliques and is a safe way to mobilize your spine. Your shoulders and arms should stay on the floor throughout but you may find to begin with that the opposite arm and shoulder come up slightly.

1 Lie on your back on the floor with your arms out to the sides at shoulder height, palms flat on the floor. Keep your knees bent. Your feet should be together and off the floor but to make this exercise easier, you can keep your feet on the floor throughout if necessary.

2 Put a cushion or pillow between your knees—this will make you keep your knees together, which is important for this exercise.

3 Tighten your abdominal muscles and remember to breathe normally—do not hold your breath.

4 Slowly bend your legs toward the floor on your right side, rolling your head to the left as you do so. Feel each part of your body peel up as you move—your buttocks, then hips, then waist and ribs. Keep going until your right knee and foot are touching the floor with your left leg lying on top.

5 Move your knees and head back to the central position.

6 Repeat this exercise on the other side with your legs toward the left side and your head to the right.

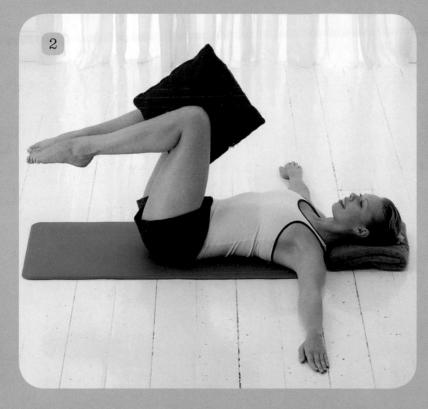

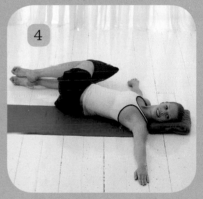

PAY ATTENTION

Don't do this exercise if you have back problems.

toe touch

This exercise helps to flatten the deep transverse muscles.

1 Lie on your back on the floor with your spine in neutral, your knees over your hips, and your feet raised, parallel to the floor.

2 Tighten your abdominal muscles by gently pulling in your navel toward your backbone—do not suck in your waist or hold your breath.

3 Slowly lower one leg until your toes touch the floor. Move your leg back to the starting position, then repeat on the other side.

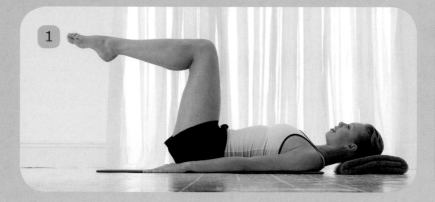

Ban the broom handle

A long-practiced exercise is to place a pole or broom handle across your shoulders and, with your arms stretched along it, twist your body vigorously from side to side in the hope that this will help to whittle your waist. This sort of exercise actually does more harm than good because it produces a ballistic twisting movement around the spine (the axis of rotation). Not only are you likely to damage your obliques, you may also stretch and tear tiny spinal ligaments. In addition, the weight of your upper body pressing down exerts extreme force on your spinal column—slipped disk, anyone? Ouch!

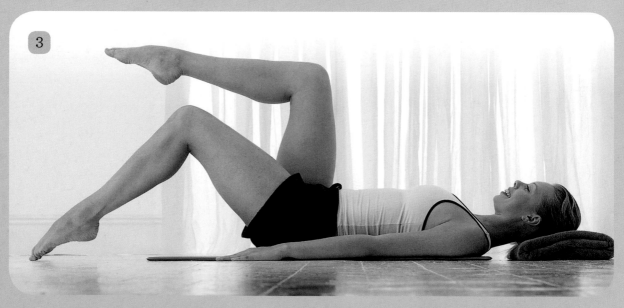

"hundreds"

This is a Pilates exercise—a system of exercise much favored by dancers—that tones the whole abdominal area. For a harder version, lift your legs off the floor and extend them (still keeping your knees slightly bent).

1 Lie on your back with your hands by your sides, hovering above the ground, palms facing downward. Keep your knees slightly bent and your feet on the floor throughout. Your spine should be in neutral. Tighten your abdominal muscles.

2 Curl your head and shoulders off the floor but keep your lower back in contact with the floor throughout. In this position, move your arms up and down, slowly breathing in and out as you do so. Breathe in for five arm movements and out for five.

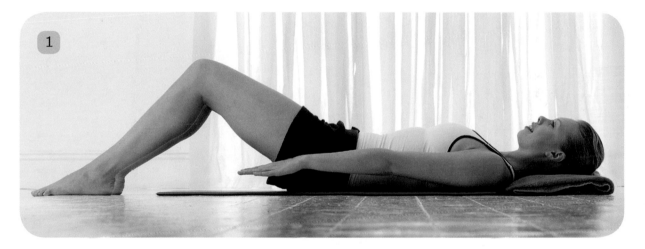

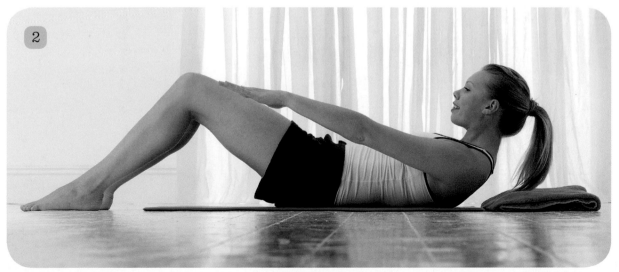

slightly harder oblique curl

You should avoid this exercise if you have neck problems.

1 Lie on your back with your spine in neutral, your knees bent, and your feet flat on the floor, hips' width apart. Put your right hand by your temple at the side of your head. Lift your left leg and rest the ankle of that leg on your right knee. Wrap your left hand around the inside of your left thigh and press your thigh outward.

2 Breathe in and tighten your abdominal muscles. Breathe out as you curl up and across to bring your right elbow toward your left knee.

3 Curl back down again, breathing in as you do so, then cross over your right leg and work the other side.

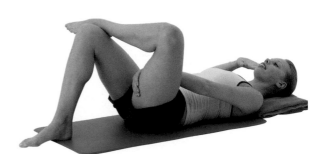

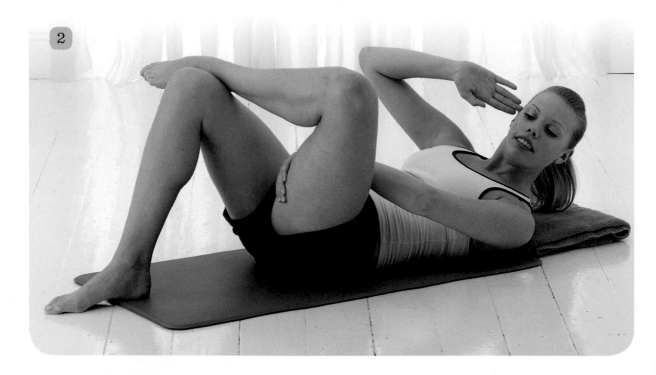

leg lift

This exercise helps to develop the deep (transverse) abdominal muscles as well as working your hamstrings (the muscles at the back of your thighs).

1 Lie on your back with your arms by your sides, palms facing downward. Keep your knees bent and feet hips' width apart, flat on the floor. Tighten your abdominal muscles.

2 Raise your left leg to the ceiling, keeping your knee slightly bent, then lower it. Then raise your right leg and lower it in the same way.

Neck support

Many people complain of neck pain when starting abdominal work. This is usually because you are using the neck muscles instead of the abdominal muscles to lift your head and shoulders. One solution is to place a towel behind your head and hold both ends taut so it supports your neck while you are curling up.

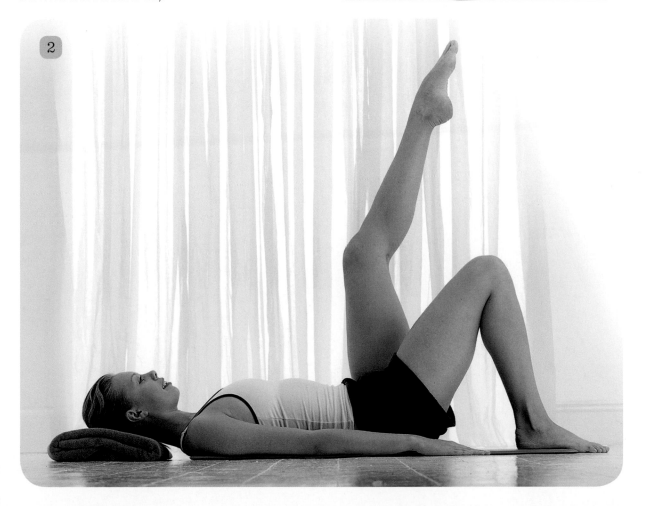

2

cooling-down exercises

Just as you need to warm up the body for exercising, you also need to cool it down after you have finished. Choose a few of the exercises shown over the next six pages, and take the time to cool down. Ideally, you should look to spend around ten minutes doing this.

lying waist stretch

This is good for giving your body an all-over general stretch, and targets the obliques, the muscles at the side of your waist.

1 Lie on the floor on your back with your knees bent and your feet flat on the floor. Keep your arms stretched out to either side. Breathe in to prepare.

2 Breathe out and pull in your abdominal muscles. Slowly bend both knees to the left while turning your head to the right.

3 Hold for a count of ten, then return to the starting position. Repeat, bending your knees to the other side.

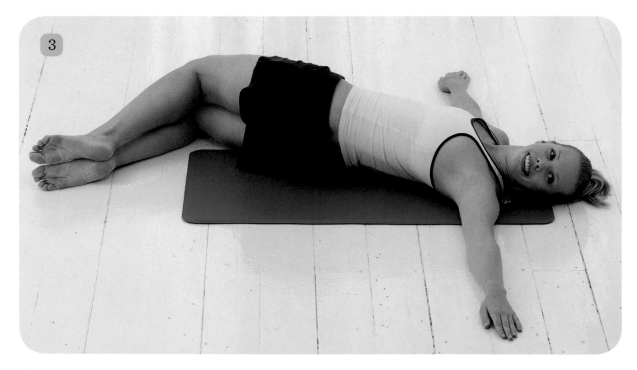

sitting body twister

You may find this stretch a little hard to perform, but this is a good way to mobilize your spine.

1 Sit on the floor with your legs straight out in front of you. Bend your right leg and cross it over your left knee.

2 Gently rotate your trunk and head toward your left as far as is comfortable, keeping your buttocks on the floor throughout.

3 Hold for a count of ten, then release and return to the starting position. Repeat on the other side.

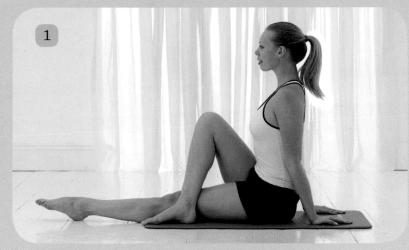

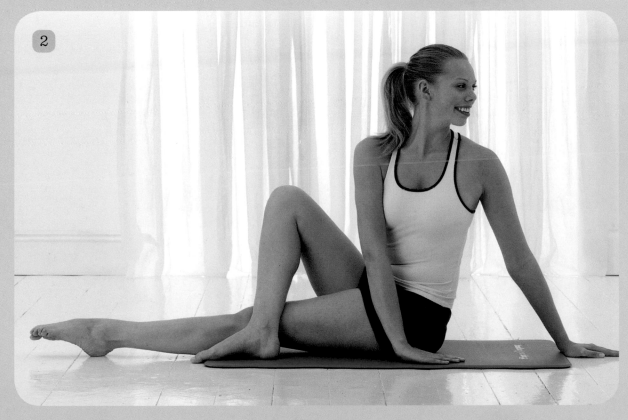

standing waist stretch

Don't lean too far over—you should feel a stretch in your obliques but it shouldn't hurt.

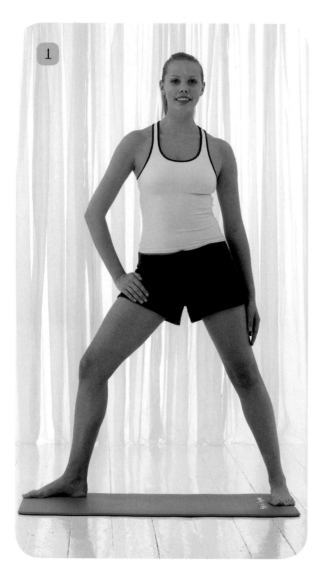

1 Stand with your legs fairly wide apart, knees soft. Turn your right foot outward and bend the knee of the right leg so that you can lunge to that side. Keep your left leg straight with the foot flat on the floor and pointing forward. Rest your right palm on your right thigh to support your body weight.

2 Lift your left arm above your head and lean toward your right side. Hold for a count of ten. Repeat on the other side.

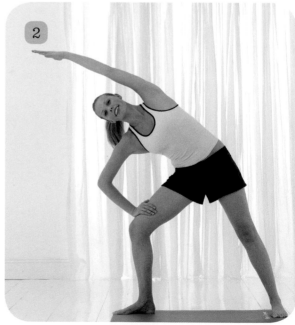

lying full body stretch

You need to find a large space on the floor to do this stretch where nothing will get in the way of you fully extending your arms and legs. This stretch will target the abdominals—the muscles across your stomach.

1 Lie flat on your back and relax. Breathe in and extend your arms outward and backward so that they meet behind your head. Try to keep your arms on the floor throughout the movement, but if this isn't possible, just keep them as low as possible.

2 Gently stretch out your body from your fingertips to your toes. Your lower back may lift from the floor a little.

3 Hold for a count of 20, then slowly release, bring your arms back down to your sides and relax.

> ### PAY ATTENTION
> If you have any back problems, keep your knees bent slightly throughout. Also, be aware that if you are unused to stretching you may feel tightness in your shoulders or cramp in your feet— in which case, relax. You will be able to hold this stretch for longer with practice.

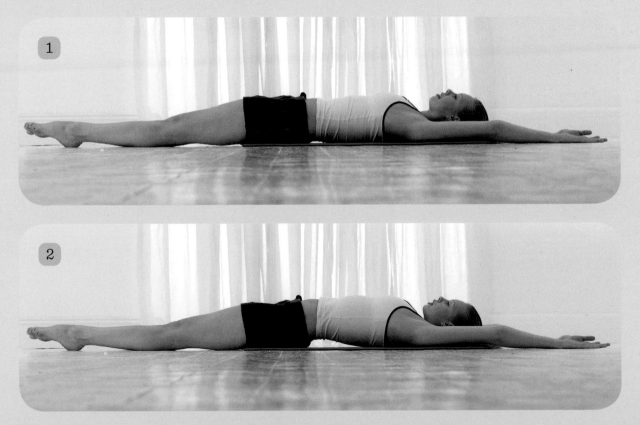

1

2

hip mobilization

You'll feel this stretch across your stomach, as you circle your hips around. It's also a great way of loosening up your hips, so it's a good stretch for starting the day.

1 Stand with feet slightly farther than hips' width apart.

2 Rest your hands on your waist and begin by slowly rotating your hips clockwise in a circular motion. Make sure you are in control of the movement and your legs stay slightly bent with feet firmly on the ground. To get the movement right, keep your back straight and try not to stick your backside out.

3 After ten seconds, repeat the same movement but this time in an counterclockwise direction.

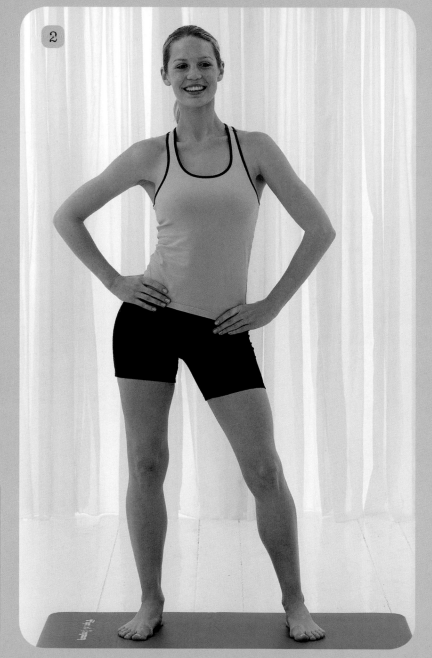

PAY ATTENTION

You should be rotating from the hips, which, when done correctly, shouldn't cause your back to arch or give you any pain. Practice this one before you start the routine—you'll be able to tell when you're doing it right by the way it feels.

twist

The twist is another great way of stretching out your obliques. This movement will help you develop long and lean muscles to support a trim waist. You're only supposed to feel a subtle stretch, so don't make the mistake of twisting around too far in order to feel a greater one.

1 Stand with feet hips' width apart. Your feet should be flat on the floor and toes should be facing forward.

2 Extend both arms out to the sides, at shoulder height.

3 Keeping your arms straight, gently rotate from the hip around to the left. Your hips and pelvis should remain facing forward.

4 Hold the position for two sets of ten seconds, until you feel the stretch in your waist. Slowly return to the starting position, then repeat on your right side.

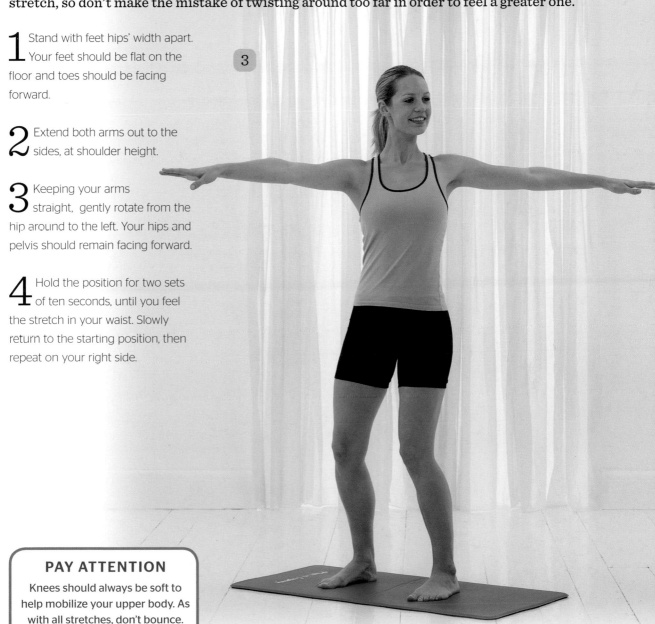

3

PAY ATTENTION
Knees should always be soft to help mobilize your upper body. As with all stretches, don't bounce.

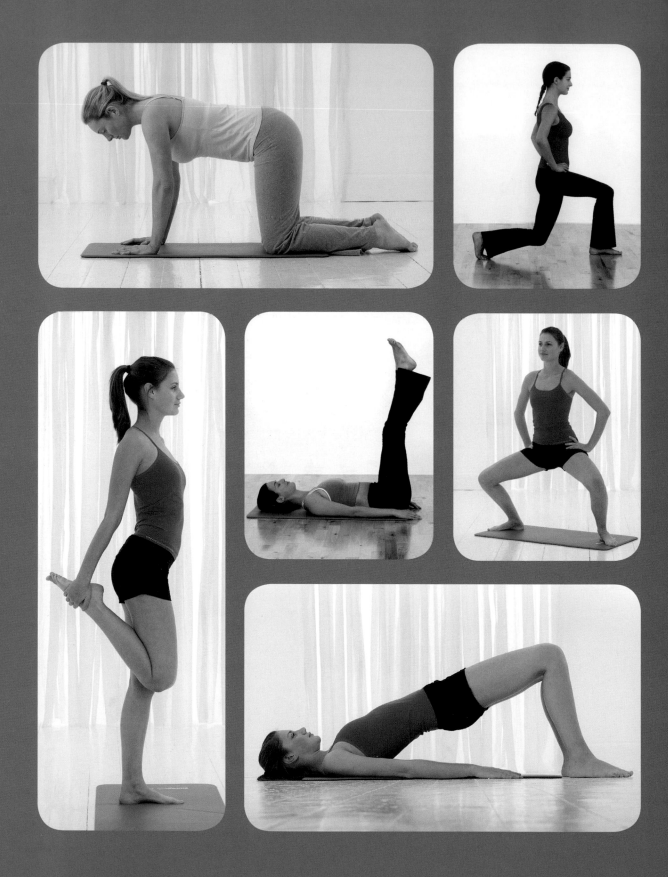

5

legs &
buttocks

If the hectic pace of daily life
prevents your thighs, hips, and
legs from getting the exercise
they need to stay in tip-top
shape, then this section is just
what you need. It features quick,
easy-to-follow exercise routines
for toning and firming the
bottom half of your body, all in
the comfort of your home!

introduction

Unless you were born with a figure to rival that of a supermodel, you probably wish your lower half was slimmer and trimmer. The trouble is that hips and thighs are often hard to target—for example, the muscles in your legs are much bigger than those in your arms, so you need to put more effort into getting results.

The benefits

General exercise, such as running, isn't always effective, so the great thing about this section is that each and every one of the exercises focuses entirely on slimming down and toning up these trouble zones.

As you can imagine, most involve a lot of leg work and it may take some time for you to build up enough strength in the legs to be able to carry out the series of exercises outlined in the 12-week plan, but with practice it will get easier.

Why not take your hip and thigh measurements before you start the plan and again when you finish? Seeing a reduction will spur you on and give you a great sense of achievement.

The muscles in the hips and thighs

It helps to have a basic understanding of the muscles you need to work on to exercise the bottom half of your body.

Buttocks: There are three buttock muscles—gluteus maximus (the biggest muscle in the body), medius, and minimus. They hold your pelvis in position, stabilize your hips, and balance the hip area. Buttock muscles help to keep you upright and pull your legs back as you walk. If you spend a lot of time sitting down, they're likely to be slack and flabby.

Hamstrings: These are three long muscles below the buttock muscles, which run from the back of the hip bone to the back of the knee. The hamstrings work with the gluteus maximus to bend your knee and rotate your hips.

Hip Flexors: A group of muscles that run from the hips to the spine and from various points along the thighbone. They include the adductors (inner thigh muscles) and abductors (outer thigh muscles). They work in opposition to the buttock muscles, helping you to move your hips and lift your thighs and knees.

Quadriceps (quads): These are four muscles that run down the front of the thigh. They enable you to extend your legs and bend your hips.

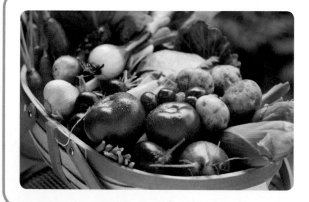

A helping hand for hips and thighs

For slimmer thighs and hips, follow a low-fat diet in addition to your toning and shaping routines.
• Trim all visible fat off meat.
• Steam or broil food instead of frying or boiling.
• Fill up with carbohydrates that release their energy slowly—for example, whole-grain pasta, rice, and cereals.
• Eat plenty of fresh fruit and vegetables.
• Drink plenty of water. This will flush out toxins from your body that can cause the appearance of dimpled flesh on your thighs.

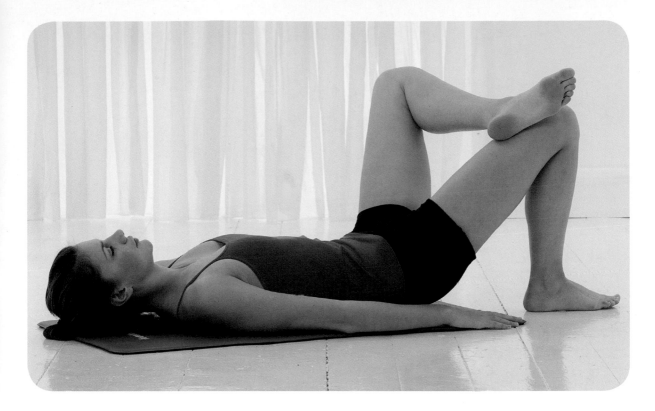

Effective exercising

Tight quads and hamstrings cause poor posture and lower back pain so it's very important to keep them in good working order. If you only ever do one type of hip and thigh exercise, make it a squat, which really hits the spot! Squats work the hip extensors, hamstrings (back of thigh muscles), and quadriceps (front of thigh muscles).

Lunges are fantastic for firming your hips and thighs, because they work the hip extensors, quadriceps, and hamstrings. They're also good exercises to help you improve your balance.

As well as tightening up your gluteals, the bridging exercises will help to stabilize your pelvis and your trunk muscles, and work your hamstrings.

Exercising on all fours makes your muscles work harder because they're working against gravity. Keep all movements smooth and controlled for best results and don't let your back sag or arch. Remember to keep your breathing steady and controlled throughout.

Do what you can!

Most of these muscle-building exercises are done as a series of repetitions. For exercises that need repeating in order to last for 30 seconds, simply do as many repetitions as you can comfortably achieve in that time. The aim of repeating exercises is to work until your muscles feel tired, and over time this will strengthen them so that they can work even harder. To make it effective, it's important that you don't stop for more than a minute between exercises. Shorter recovery periods result in better muscles all around and improved muscle endurance. So keep going!

What you'll need

For this section, you'll need a nonslip mat or pair of sneakers, a chair, and a platform to step up onto or a sturdy bottom stair on a staircase. Don't forget to warm up before you begin and cool down when you finish. Now let's get started.

warming-up exercises

It is always essential to warm up before undertaking any form of exercise. Choose a couple of the exercises shown over the next few pages and spend a little time warming up. You should allow around ten minutes for this, and alternate them so you don't get bored.

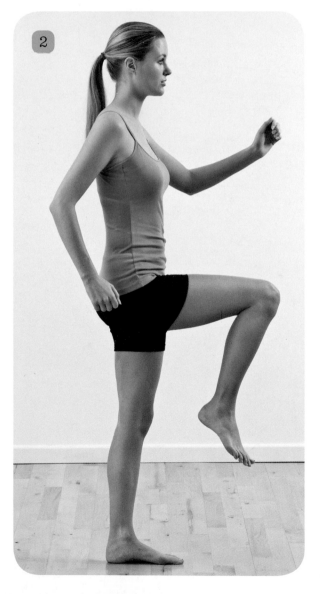

marching on the spot

This is a very easy and safe way to gently start warming up your body.

1 Stand with good posture, by having your feet hip-width apart, knees soft, stomach pulled in, and shoulders pulled back. Starting from this position ensures you are exercising in a safe manner. Begin marching on the spot.

2 Be sure to keep your upper body straight and your stomach muscles pulled in. Aim to gradually lift your knees to hip height and then bend your arms and swing them back and forth as you would do if you were walking fast.

3 Do this for between two to three minutes until you feel fully warmed up. Alternatively, you can warm up by going for a brisk walk around the block.

hip circles

Try this exercise to warm up your pelvic muscles. Keep your torso still—only your pelvis should be moving.

1 Stand up straight with your knees slightly bent, feet hips' width apart, and your hands resting on your hips.

2 Gently draw in your navel toward your spine to tighten your abdominal muscles. Do not suck in your waist or hold your breath—this movement should feel light and subtle.

3 Slowly circle your pelvis to the right so that you are rotating in a full circle.

4 Repeat to the right, then circle to the left

Exercise tip

Loosening up the body before exercising is important because it prepares the muscles and joints for the workout and also increases the heart rate, causing the blood to pump faster around the body. Consequently, the harder the muscles work, the more beneficial the exercise will be.

However, do not try to push any of the moves too far, too soon. Always keep the principles in mind and always think "quality."

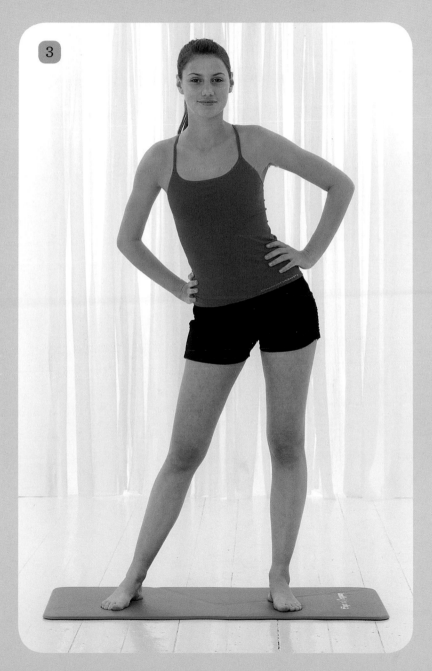

knee bends

This exercise loosens the hip flexor muscles and helps warm up all the leg muscles. Don't lock your knees as you do this, and bend only as far as is comfortable.

1 Stand with one hand resting on a support, such as a high-backed chair or a table, your feet hips' width apart and slightly turned out. Tighten your abdominal muscles.

2 Slowly bend your knees and lower your hips, then straighten up again. Use your buttock and leg muscles to lower and straighten.

3 Repeat ten times.

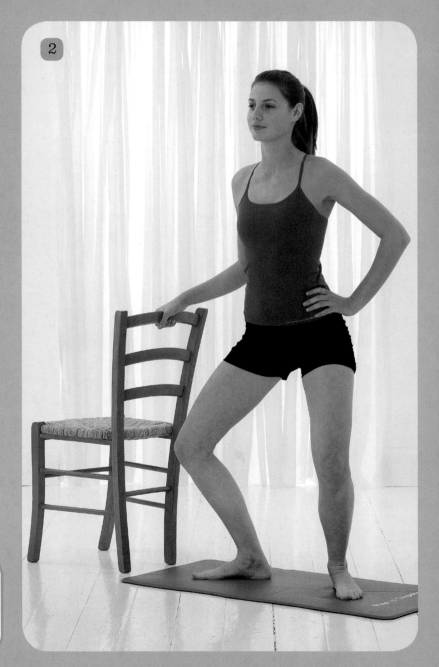

PAY ATTENTION
Never point your toes inward while exercising—this can damage your knees.

leg swings

This exercise warms up the hip joints and increases blood circulation. Don't swing your legs too high (about 45 degrees is high enough), and keep the movements controlled and flowing.

1 Stand with one hand resting on a support, such as a high-backed chair or a table, and balance on one leg with the knee slightly bent. Tighten your stomach muscles to protect your back.

2 Gently swing your other leg forward and backward. Keep your hips still as your leg moves from back to front. Swing up to 20 times on one leg, then swap sides and swing on the other leg.

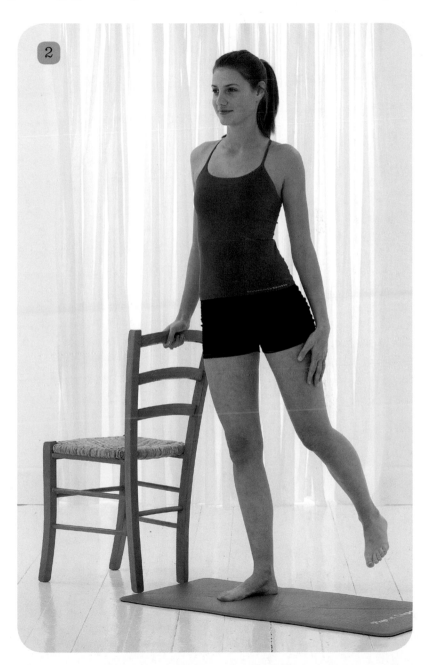

PAY ATTENTION

Ensure that you don't arch your back as your leg swings behind you.

standing knee lift

This exercise mobilizes the quadriceps and the hip flexors at the front of your body.

1 Stand up straight with your left hand on a chair to balance you.

2 Tighten your abdominal muscles.

3 Pull up your right knee so that your foot is parallel to your left knee.

4 Release and repeat on the other leg.

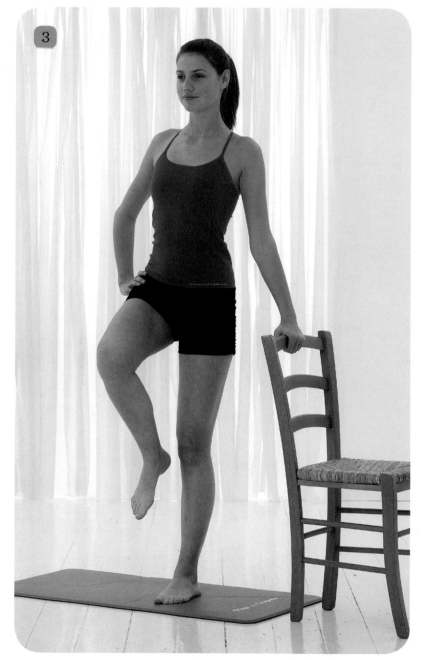

standing leg circles

This exercise warms up the buttock muscles by lifting and drawing them together.

1 Stand up straight with good posture with your knees soft and legs hips' width apart. For balance, hold onto a chair.

2 Tighten your abdominal muscles by gently pulling in your navel toward your backbone.

3 Lift your left leg a few inches off the floor and gently circle it one way, then the other.

4 Return to the starting position and repeat on the other leg

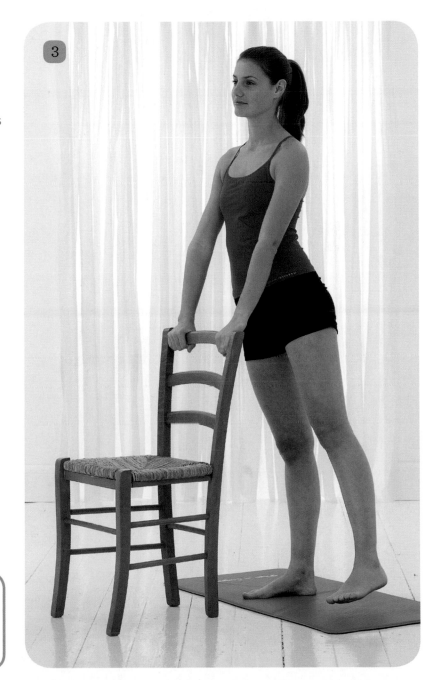

Exercise tip

Make sure you use a straight-backed, sturdy chair when exercising—not one on wheels.

introductory exercises

These first-stage exercises are aimed at beginners, so you should find them relatively easy to start with, allowing you to become more involved as you progress. If you find any of the exercises a bit too difficult, feel free to replace them with something else of the same level.

basic squat

Targeting the buttocks and tops of the thighs, this easy exercise is great for toning up those trouble spots. Remember to keep your knees soft (slightly bent) throughout.

1 Stand up with good posture, your feet hips' width apart and your hands on your hips.

2 Tighten your abdominal muscles by gently pulling your navel toward your spine.

3 Bend your knees and squat as if you were going to sit down. Only squat as far as is comfortable and without losing your balance.

4 Return to the standing position by pushing through your heels, keeping your knees slightly bent as you do so.

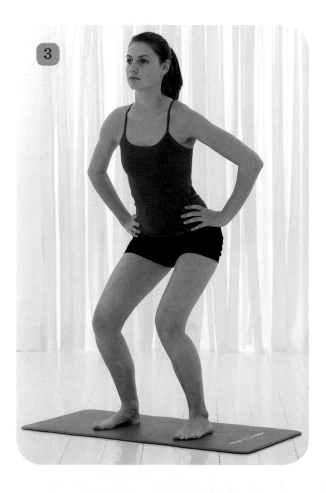

Exercise tip

If you only ever do one type of hip and thigh exercise, make it a squat, which really hits the spot! Squats work the hip extensors, hamstrings (back of thigh muscles), and quadriceps (front of thigh muscles). Tight quads and hamstrings cause poor posture and lower back pain so it's very important to keep them in good working order.

buttock walking

This exercise is wonderful for keeping your backside trim and strengthening the buttock muscles. The floor is a good option because a hard surface is more taxing, but beware of carpet burn, or splinters from old wooden floors.

1 Sit up straight with your legs stretched out in front of you. Cross your arms so that your hands are resting on your shoulders.

2 Breathe in and lengthen your spine. Breathe out, and breathe normally as you "walk" forward on your buttocks—ten steps forward, ten steps back to form one repetition. Repeat as often as you can.

PAY ATTENTION
Be careful not to overarch your back on this one.

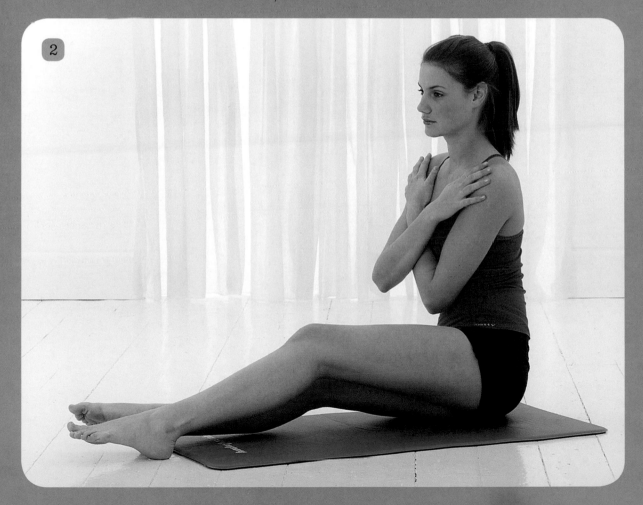

standing calf raises

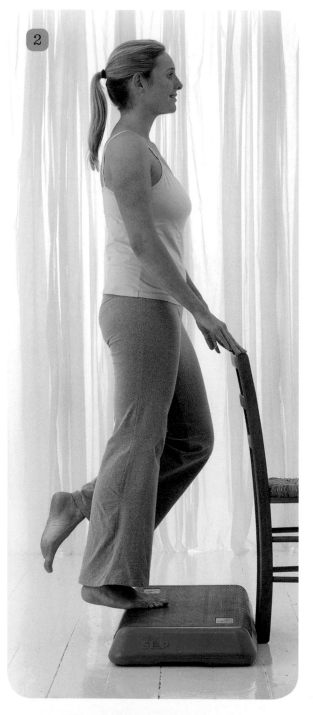

The calf muscles are hard to target, although studies have shown that walking in high heels can help to tone them up! To get really sexy, shapely calves, we recommend you try this exercise instead.

1 Stand with both feet near the edge of a raised object, such as a stair or a big chunky book. Place the ball of your right foot on the edge of the raised object, letting your heel extend off the edge.

2 Hold onto a wall or a chair for support and, lifting your left leg into the air slightly by bending at the knee, gently let your right heel drop down until you feel the stretch in your calf. Keep your back straight, your head up, and your right leg straight.

3 Rise up onto your right toe as high as you can and hold for a second while flexing the calf muscle.

4 Carefully return to the starting position, then repeat with the left leg.

PAY ATTENTION
Make sure that you don't slip off the raised object by carefully controlling the move. If that means you have to do fewer reps on each foot during the exercise, so be it.

stepping

This is a great exercise if you like "feeling the burn." Stepping up onto a stair forces the glutes (the muscles in the buttocks) to squeeze and contract, so will help create a pert backside.

1 Stand at the buttocks of the stairs or in front of a big chunky book. Rest your hands on your hips or let them rest by your side.

2 Step up onto the step with your left leg and let your right leg follow.

3 Step down off the step with your left leg and let the right leg follow.

4 Repeat, starting with the right leg. You should be able to manage around 15 or more during the 30 seconds.

> ### PAY ATTENTION
> Do this barefoot or wear a good pair of sneakers instead of slippery socks for this exercise so that you don't slip off the step. Plus, don't rush the move.

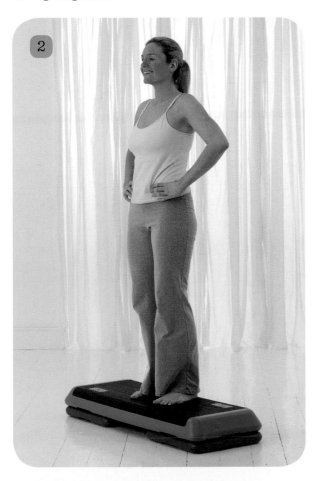

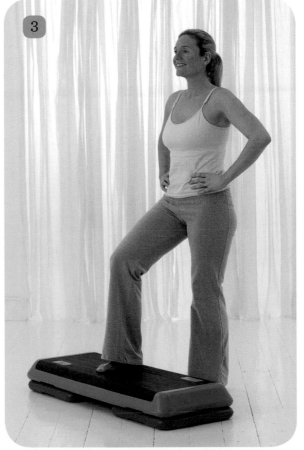

bridge squeeze

This buttock-clenching exercise makes the gluteus maximus work to support your back. If you feel a strong contraction in your hamstrings or any strain in your lower back, then you are not using your buttock muscles properly.

1 Lie on your back with your knees bent and feet slightly apart.

2 Tighten your abdominal muscles by gently drawing in your navel toward your spine—which will protect your back muscles.

3 Curl your backside off the floor, lifting your pelvis until your knees, hips, and chest are in line.

4 Hold this for a count of ten, squeezing your buttock muscles to support the bridge position. Release and repeat.

Exercise tip

As well as tightening up your gluteals, this bridging exercise will help to stabilize your pelvis and your trunk muscles, and work your hamstrings. Be careful not to overarch your back or let it sag, and remember to keep your breathing steady and controlled throughout.

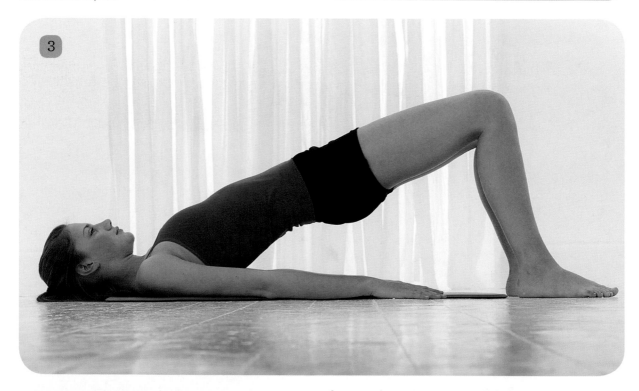

3

kneeling kickback

This works your quadriceps.

1 Get down on all fours and pull in your stomach muscles to protect your back.

2 Raise your right leg off the floor, and with your knee bent, bring it into your body, then stretch it out backward so that it is in line with your body with the foot flexed.

3 Pull the leg back in and take it back out again. Do all your repetitions on one leg, then repeat using the other leg.

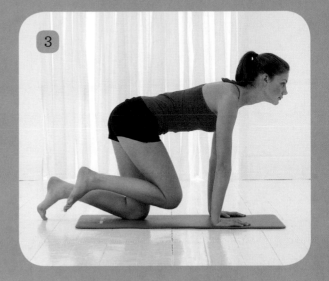

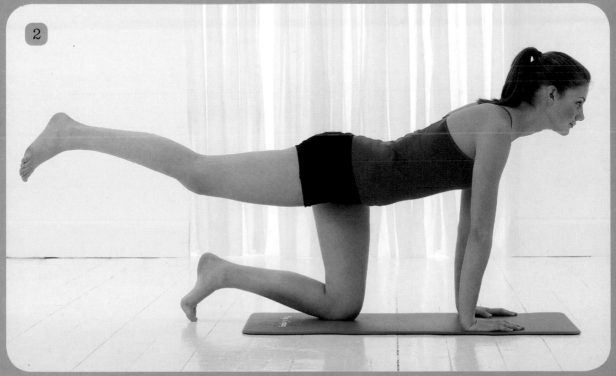

superman

You need to have a good sense of balance to do this exercise, so if you don't get it right first time, be patient. It's great for increasing stability and endurance in the joints, as well as working the core muscles in your thighs.

1 Get down on the floor on all fours, then pull in your abdominal muscles.

2 Extend your right arm out in front of you and your left leg out behind you, keeping it as straight as you can without locking your elbow or knee. Engage your abdominal muscles to help prevent your back from arching—it will reduce any risk of injury. You will feel the muscles working in the thigh of your extended leg. If you want to increase the effects, point your toes—it will make you tense your muscles even harder. Keep your head and neck in line with your back to make sure you're not twisting your neck.

3 Slowly return to the start position and repeat with the opposite leg and arm.

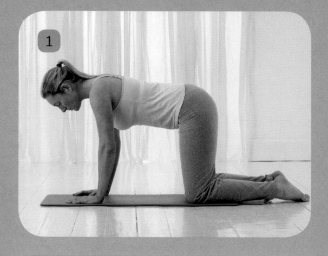

PAY ATTENTION
Do this on soft carpet or a padded exercise mat, so you don't hurt your knees.

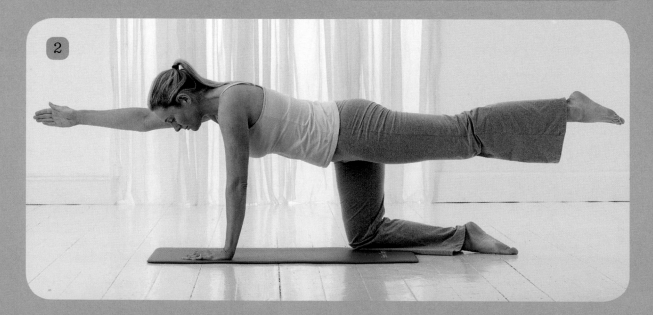

inner thigh lift

These side-lying exercises work your inner thigh muscles (abductors). Remember to keep your spine in neutral and your stomach muscles tightened throughout.

1 Lie on one side with your hips facing forward and your body in a straight line. Prop yourself up on your elbow with your head resting on your hand and place the other hand on the floor in front of you for support.

2 Tighten your stomach muscles by gently drawing in your navel toward your spine to protect your back.

3 Bend your top leg so that the knee touches the floor in front of you.

4 Raise the bottom extended leg, keeping the knee soft (slightly bent), then lower.

5 Do all your repetitions on one side, then repeat them on the other side of your body.

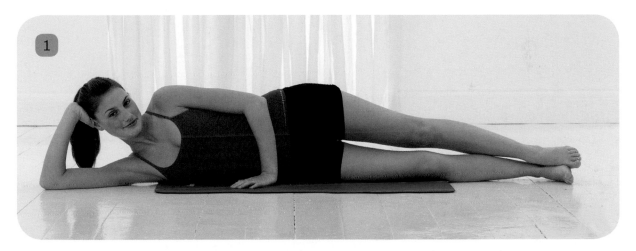

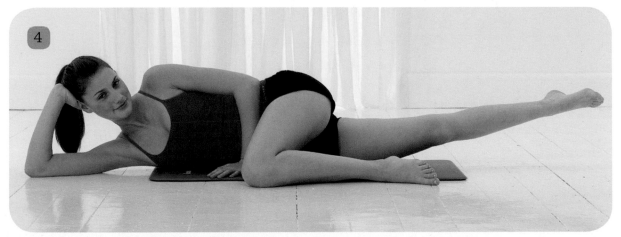

outer thigh lift

Make sure you perform each move slowly and in a controlled way to really work the muscles. You don't have to tense your buttocks as you do this, but it's good to work your gluteals whenever you can.

1 Lie on your right side with your body in a straight line and your thighs and feet together. Prop yourself up with your right arm and rest your left hand on the floor in front of you. Tighten your stomach muscles by drawing your navel in toward your spine—this will help to protect your back.

2 Bend both knees. Lift up the top leg, then lower, squeezing your buttocks together as you raise and lower your leg.

3 Do all your repetitions on one side, then repeat on the other side of your body.

PAY ATTENTION
Keep the knee of the extended leg soft (slightly bent).

2

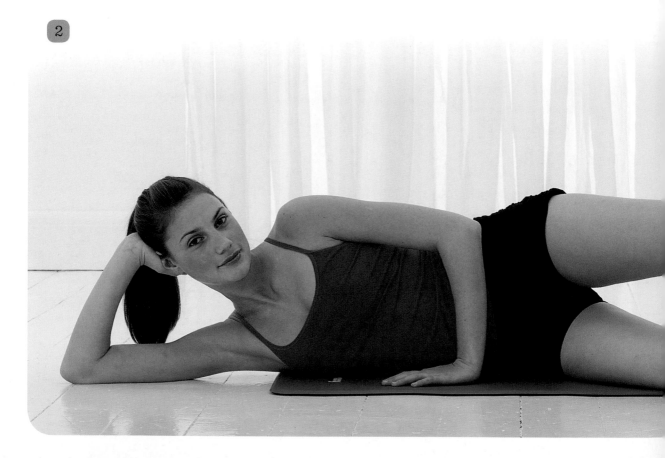

straight leg outer thigh lift

A variation of the outer thigh lift.

1 Lie on your side with your lower leg bent and your top leg straight but with the knee soft, not locked. Your body should be in a straight line and your thighs and knees together. Prop yourself up on your elbow with your head resting on your hand and place the other hand in front of you for support. Keep your stomach muscles pulled in to protect your back.

2 Raise your top leg, then lower it, squeezing your buttock muscles as you do so. If you are in the correct position, you shouldn't be able to lift your leg more than 45 degrees.

3 Do all your repetitions on one side, then repeat them on the other side of your body.

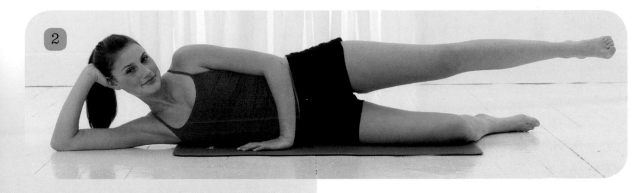

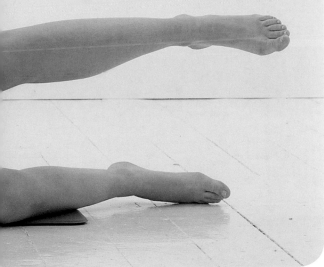

Keeping up your motivation

All too often people start a new exercise routine burning with enthusiasm, only for it to peter out very quickly to the point where they can't be bothered to do anything at all. When you start your exercise program, be realistic about how and when you can do it. You need to set aside a regular slot for your routine so it becomes a natural and automatic part of your everyday routine. But if you do miss several days, don't get disheartened and give up—a little exercise even on a very irregular basis is still better than nothing at all.

advanced exercises

Now that you've worked through the introductory exercises and are feeling more confident and fitter, you can progress to this second series of exercises. As before, if you find any particular exercises too difficult, feel free to replace them with something else from this level.

wide squat

Wide squats are great for toning your inner thigh muscles and the front and back of the thighs. Try not to wobble.

1 Stand up with good posture, your feet wide apart and your toes turned out. Keep your hands on your hips.

2 Tighten your abdominal muscles by gently pulling your navel toward your spine.

3 Bend your knees and lower your backside as if you were going to sit down.

4 Go as low as you can without wobbling forward. Return to a standing position by pushing through your heels, keeping your knees slightly bent as you do so.

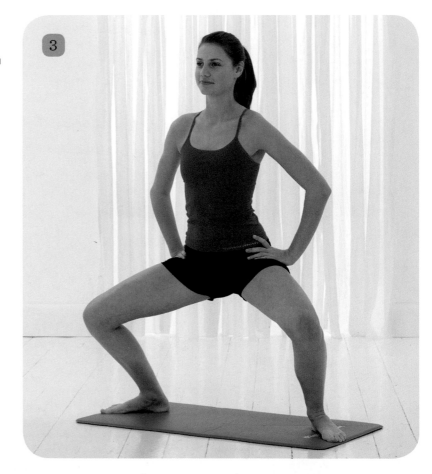

lunge

The farther you step forward in this exercise, the harder your muscles will be worked.

1 Stand with your hands on your hips and your feet parallel and hips' width apart. Brace your abdominal muscles.

2 Take a big step forward, keeping your weight evenly balanced between both legs.

3 Bend both knees as far as is comfortable so that you lower your torso down, then return to the starting position.

4 Repeat on the other leg.

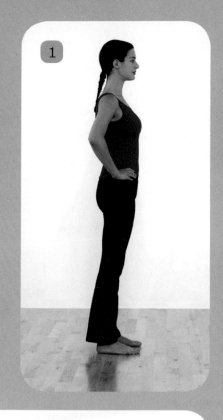

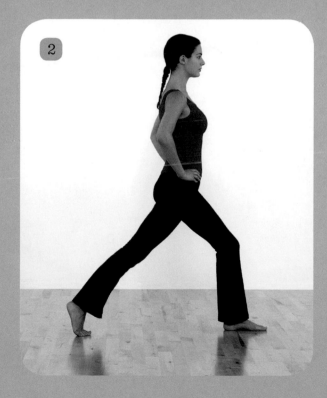

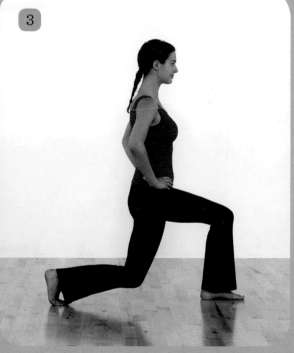

double knee bends

This exercise, which strengthens your thighs, calves, and buttocks, will help you achieve the sculpted legs of a dancer.

1 Stand with your legs a little wider than shoulders' width apart and your feet slightly turned out. Rest your hands on the back of a chair to help you balance.

2 Tighten your abdominal muscles to protect your lower back.

3 Slowly press your knees out and lower yourself down. You should feel this in your buttocks and the back of your thighs.

4 Return to standing, then tense your buttocks, squeeze your inner thigh muscles and rise up onto your toes. Return to the start position.

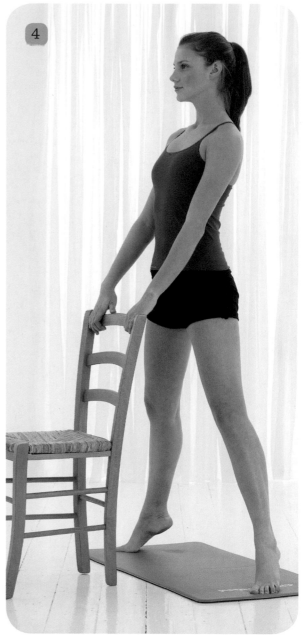

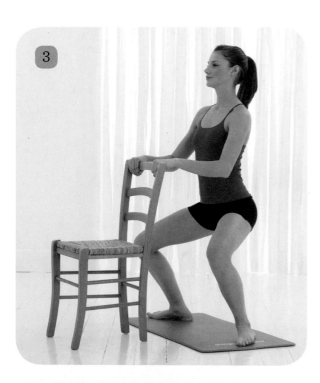

front leg raise

This exercise strengthens and tones the front of your thighs (quadriceps) and increases your hip flexibility. It also helps with your balance.

1 Stand up straight with your feet together and hold onto the back of a chair sideways with your left hand to balance. Tighten your stomach muscles.

2 With your left leg slightly bent, raise your right leg out in front of you as far as is comfortable. Hold for a count of three.

3 Lower your leg, then do all your repetitions on that leg. Repeat on the other leg.

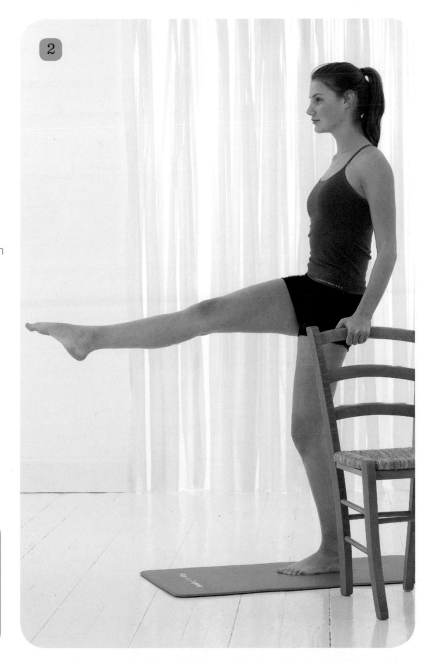

Exercise tip

These traditional ballet exercises give a great workout to the legs and buttocks. Keep your movements controlled and flowing.

scissors

You will feel a stretch in your hamstrings as you perform this exercise but the main aim is to keep your pelvis, hips, and spine still and maintain abdominal tension throughout.

1 Lie on your back with both legs raised, toes pointing to the ceiling and knees slightly bent.

2 Keep your spine in neutral and set your abdominal muscles.

3 Slowly lower your left leg down toward the floor, still keeping your torso in alignment. From this position, change the position of your legs in a scissoring action.

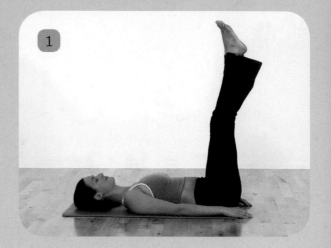

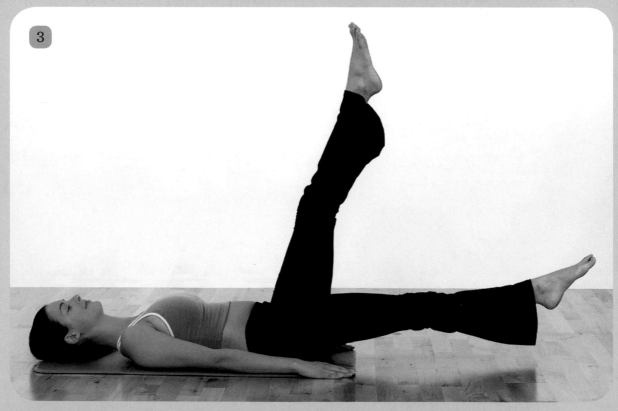

one leg knee bends

These will strengthen your buttocks, thigh muscles, and calves.

1 Stand up with good posture with your right side to the back of a chair and hold onto it for support. Lift and bend your right leg backward so that the knee faces forward and your foot is pointing out behind you in line with your knee.

2 Tighten your abdominal muscles to protect your back.

3 Slowly rise up onto the toes of your left foot. Hold for a count of two.

4 Slowly come back down again onto your left foot.

5 Now bend your left knee, bringing the kneecap directly over your foot.

6 Straighten up and repeat on the same leg, then do this exercise on the other leg.

PAY ATTENTION
Don't let your backside stick out.

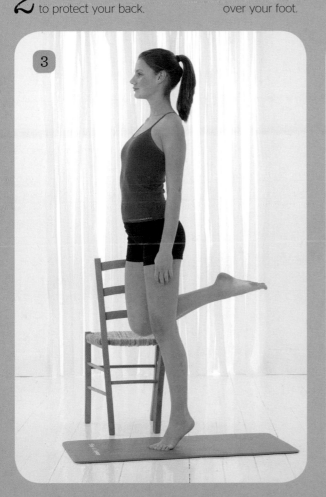

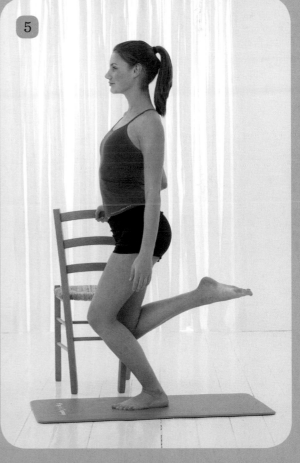

leg lift

This is a lateral thigh raise that works the outer thigh muscles (hip abductors).

1 To start, kneel in the "box" position (on all fours) and keep your back straight. Tighten your abdominal muscles to support your back.

2 Lift your right leg out to the side—you will feel the muscles at the side of the thigh and hip working to lift your leg. Hold for a count of two.

3 Slowly lower your leg to the start position. Do all your repetitions on one leg, then repeat using the other leg.

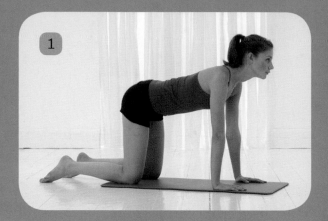

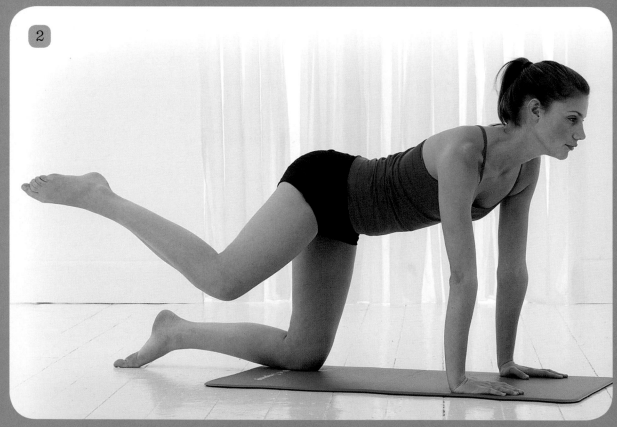

straight leg inner thigh lift

This is a harder exercise, which tones your inner thigh muscles.

1 Lie on your side with your hips facing forward and your body in a straight line. Prop yourself up on your elbow with your head resting on your hand and place the other hand on the floor in front of you for support.

2 Tighten your stomach muscles by gently drawing in your navel toward your spine to protect your back.

3 Bend your top leg and place the foot flat on the floor just above the knee of the extended leg.

4 Raise your extended leg off the floor as far as you can (this won't be very far), then lower.

5 Do all your repetitions on one side, then repeat on the other leg.

> **PAY ATTENTION**
> Don't raise your bottom leg too high
> —or you'll overextend the muscles.

> **Don't exercise if…**
> • you are feeling unwell—your body will need all its strength to fight off any infection.
> • you have an injury—you might make things worse.
> • you have an ongoing medical condition or are on medication—consult your doctor first.
> • you've just had a big meal.
> • you've been drinking alcohol.

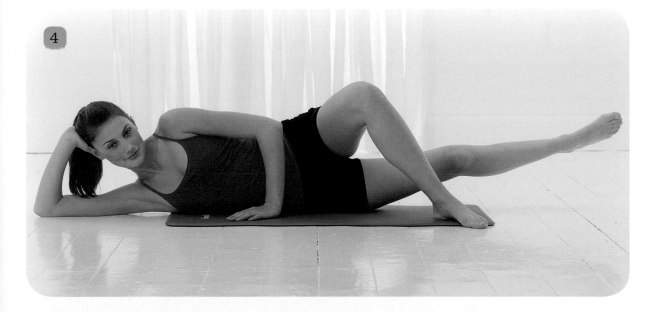

one leg buttock clencher

This is a harder exercise that will really work your gluteals.

1 Lie on your back with your knees bent and your feet flat on the floor, slightly apart. Keep your arms by your sides, palms facing downward.

2 Place your left foot on to your right knee. Tighten your abdominal muscles to support your back.

3 Press your lower back down into the floor and gently tilt your pelvis forward so that the pubic bone rises. Lift your hips off the floor and squeeze your buttock muscles, then release.

4 Do all your repetitions on one leg, then repeat on the other leg.

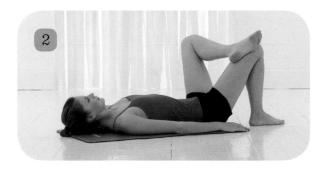

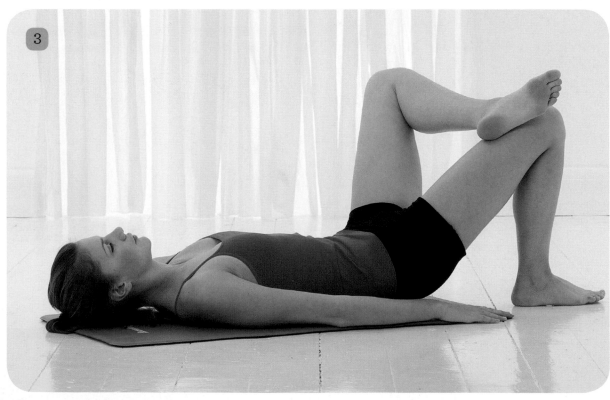

bridge with leg lift

Lifting one leg strengthens the muscles at the back of the buttocks and thighs while increasing balance and control in your stabilizing muscles.

1 Lie on your back with your knees bent and feet slightly apart, and your arms at your sides.

2 Tighten your abdominal muscles by gently drawing in your navel toward your spine.

3 Curl your backside off the floor, lifting your pelvis until your knees, hips, and chest are in line.

4 Extend one leg, lift it level with the knee, then lower to the floor. Do all your repetitions on one leg, then repeat on the other leg.

Controlling your movements

Make sure that all exercises are performed slowly, carefully, and with your full attention. You really do need to concentrate on what you're doing and think about how your body is responding to any exercise.

If an action hurts or you do it too quickly, then you're not doing it properly. Movements should flow in a gentle, controlled manner. This enables your muscles to stretch naturally.

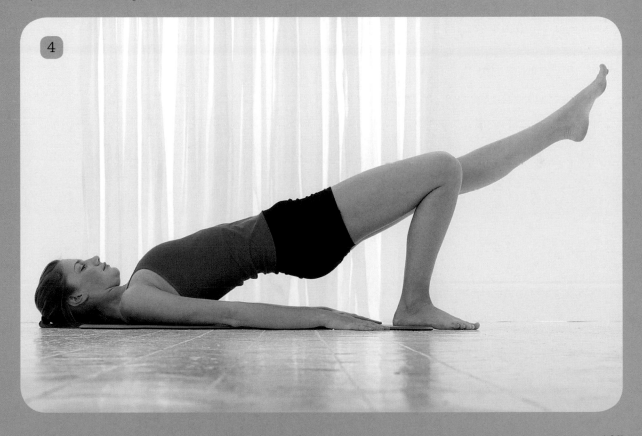

4

cooling-down exercises

Just as you need to warm up the body for exercising, you also need to cool it down after you have finished. Choose a few of the exercises shown over the next eight pages, and take the time to cool down. Ideally, you should look to spend around ten minutes doing this.

lying quad stretch

The quadriceps muscles are found at the front of your thighs and are often referred to as the "quads."

1 Lie prone (face down) on the floor. Bend one knee and take hold of the foot of that leg with your hand and gently pull the foot toward your buttock.

2 Press your hip down toward the floor, which will ensure you stretch fully the rectus femoris (the quadriceps muscle that crosses the hip joint).

3 Hold the stretch for a count of 20, then release and repeat on the other leg.

Top tips for stretching

- Only stretch warm muscles.
- Slowly ease the muscles into position.
- Never bounce into position.
- Do not overstretch—mild discomfort is acceptable but if it hurts, you should stop.
- Breathe freely to enable blood to flow to the muscles—do not hold your breath.

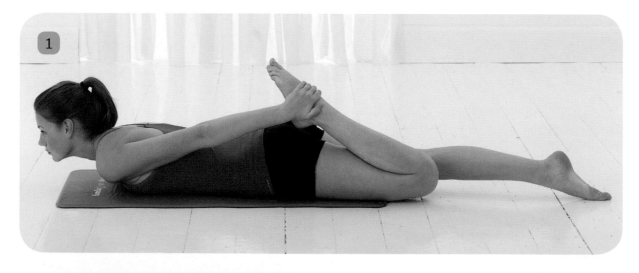

standing quad stretch

Depending on how flexible you are, this stretch may feel quite hard to do at first, but it quickly becomes easier.

1 Stand up straight with your feet hips' width apart and your knees soft (slightly bent). Tighten your stomach muscles to protect your back.

2 Bend your left leg up behind you and hold your foot or ankle with your left hand.

3 Hold for 20 seconds, then release and repeat on the other side.

4 Repeat twice more on each leg.

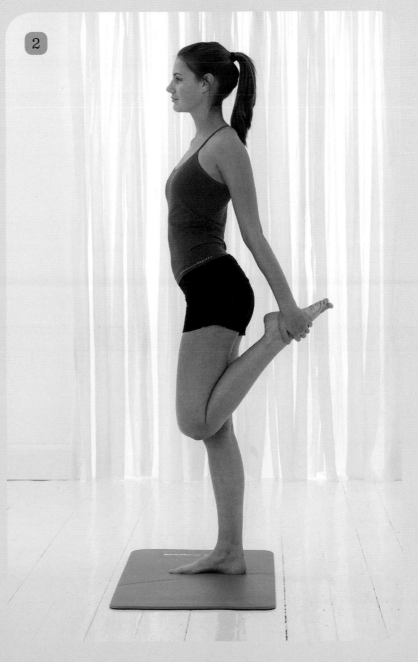

Start marching!

Before you begin your stretches, it is a good idea to march on the spot for a couple of minutes to gently bring your heart rate and body temperature back to their preexercise state. Do this by gradually easing your march to a slow pace and then coming to a halt.

standing hamstring stretch

The hamstrings are the muscles running up the backs of the thighs to your backside. It's common for people have with tight hamstrings, especially if they do a lot of sport, which is why it's great to stretch them out.

1 Stand up straight with your knees hips' width apart and your knees soft (slightly bent).

2 Extend one foot forward so that it is pointing in front of you with the weight resting on its heel. Tighten your stomach muscles to protect your back.

3 Rest your hands on the thigh of the bent leg to support your body weight.

4 Bend forward from the hip and feel the stretch in the back of the thigh of the straight leg.

5 Hold for 20 seconds, then release and repeat on the other side.

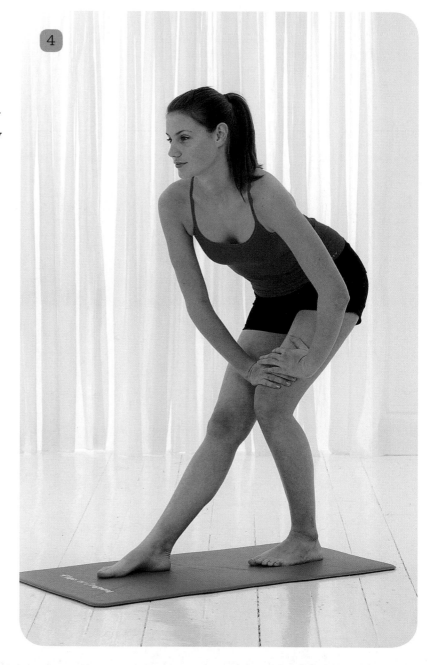

lying hamstring stretch

If you don't stretch, tight hamstrings can cause the hips and pelvis to rotate backward, resulting in bad posture.

1 Lie on your back with your knees bent and your feet resting flat on the floor.

2 Lift one leg and grasp the back of the thigh with your hands.

3 Gently pull that leg toward your chest as far as is comfortable. Repeat on the other leg.

Train your brain

Use your mind to help you get the most from your workout. Focus on what you are doing correctly. As you are exercising, tell yourself how well you are doing. Think of each muscle contracting and stretching as you do your routine. This can make you do even better, whereas concentrating on what you are doing wrong sets you up to fail. You can even use visualizations to convince yourself that your body is becoming fitter and more toned!

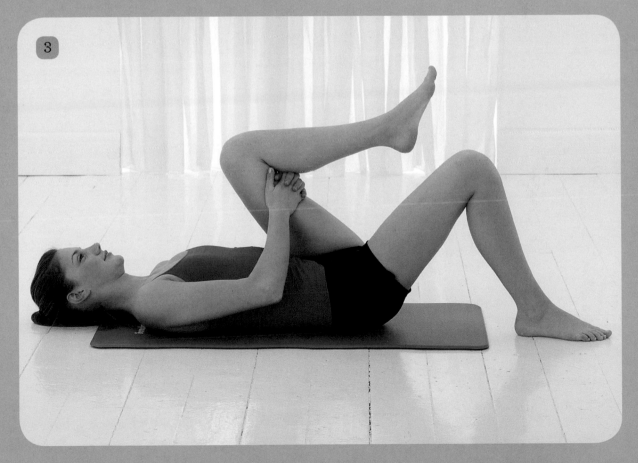

lying buttock stretch

This will stretch your buttocks and your outside thigh muscles.

1 Lie on your back and bend your legs. Cross your right ankle over your left knee and lift your left leg off the floor. You will feel a stretch on the outside thigh and buttock of your left leg.

2 Take hold of your left thigh with both hands and slowly draw the left knee in toward you. You will feel the stretch intensify.

3 Hold the stretch for a count of ten. Release and repeat on the other leg.

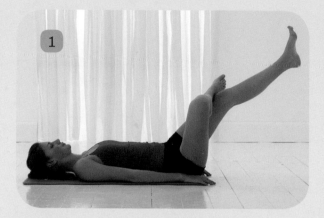

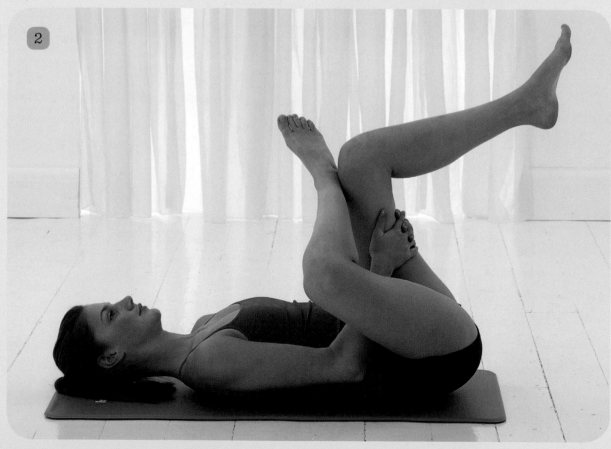

push-off calf stretch

You usually see joggers doing this stretch before a big run—that's because it's a really good way of performing a controlled calf stretch that targets the gastrocnemius muscle (the big muscle at the back of the calf). To get the best stretch possible, make sure your full weight is shifted toward the wall.

1 Stand at arm's length from the wall, with your feet shoulders' width apart.

2 Extend your right leg out in front of you and bend your right knee.

3 Place the palms of your hands, at shoulder height, flat against the wall.

4 Take one step back with your left leg and, keeping it straight, press your heel firmly into the floor. You should feel the stretch in the calf of your left leg. Keep your hips facing the wall and your rear leg and spine in a straight line.

5 Hold the stretch for two sets of ten seconds, then repeat with the other leg.

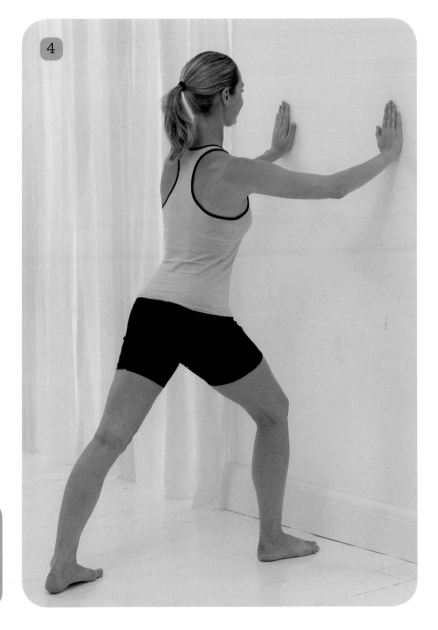

PAY ATTENTION
If you want to feel a greater stretch, simply move your extended leg a little bit farther away from the wall.

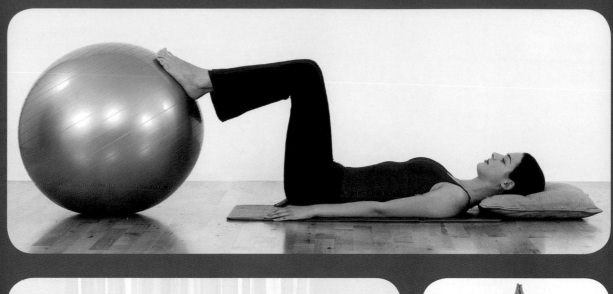

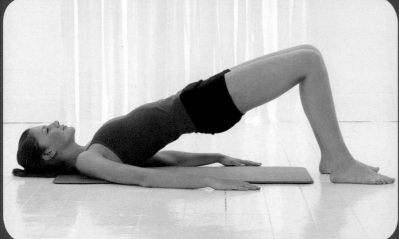

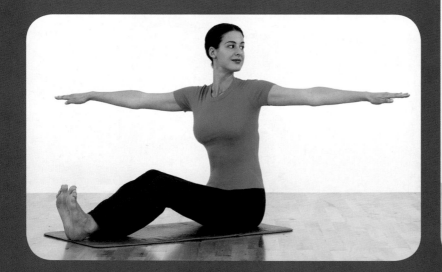

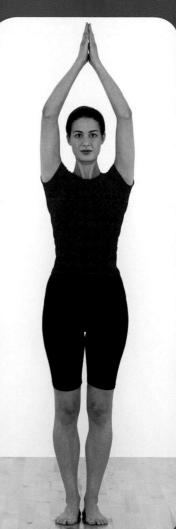

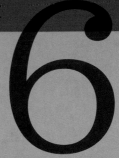

core stability

Core stability is the effective use of the core muscles to help stabilize the spine, allowing your limbs to move more freely. The positive effects of good core stability include reducing the likelihood of injury, better posture, increased agility and flexibility, and improved coordination.

introduction

Core training is a workout that strengthens your body from the inside out by concentrating on the muscles that form your "core." The core of your body is simply what's between the shoulders and hips—basically, the trunk and pelvis. Core training reeducates these muscles to make them more effective.

The core is a crucial group of muscles, not only for sports, but for normal daily activities as well, because it comes into play just about every time you move. The core acts to produce force (for example, during lifting), it stabilizes the body to permit other musculature to produce force (for example, during running) and it's also called upon to transfer energy (for example, during jumping).

This is why it is so important that your core is strong. Once you have learned how to strengthen your core, your lower abdominal muscles will be drawn in toward the spine and help you sit up straight. Your balance and coordination will be improved, and, most important of all, the stability these muscles bring will help keep your spine healthy and flexible.

What is core stability?

Core stability is the effective use of the core muscles to help stabilize the spine, allowing your limbs to move more freely. Good core stability means you can keep your midsection rigid without forces, such as gravity, affecting your movements. The positive effects of this include reducing the chance of injury, better posture, increased agility and flexibility, and improved coordination.

Core stability can be increased by developing trunk fitness, which is necessary for everyday life not just for sport. To pick up a child, for example, requires a core strength in order to not only lift the child but also to do it in a safe way that avoids you injuring yourself. To really

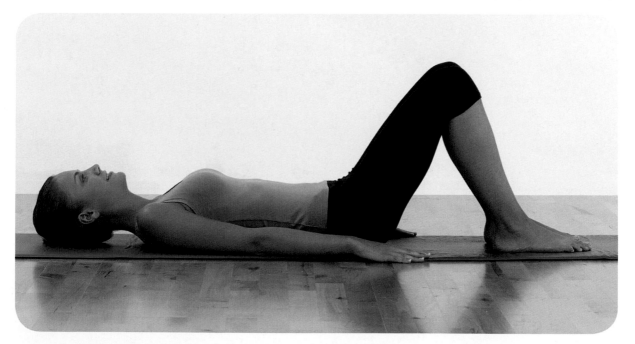

capture the benefits of core strength, including better alignment, balance, and functional movement (as well as flat abs), it is necessary to work the deep, underlying abdominal and back musculature.

Core muscles

The muscles you need to know about for improving your core stability are those that are arranged around your torso, or trunk.

The trunk muscles fall into two categories: inner (mainly responsible for stabilization) and outer (mainly responsible for movement). The inner unit muscles include the transversus abdominis, diaphragm, multifidus, and pelvic floor; the outer unit includes the obliques and spinal erectors. The inner and outer units work together to create spinal stability and enable subsequent movement.

How to train your core

The core muscles should be loaded with resistance, and challenged in a variety of ways—by lateral (side) flexion, bending forward and backward, and rotation. If strength and muscle development is the goal, hundreds of repetitions are not necessary. Core strength should be developed gradually to decrease the risk of injury. When starting out on a core training program, you need to progress properly:

• Start with the easiest movements and progress to more difficult movements.

• Perform all movements in a slow and controlled manner until coordination, strength, and confidence permit higher-speed movements.

• To increase the complexity and muscle demands of the exercises, many moves can be performed lying prone (face down) or supine (on your back) on an exercise ball or other unstable platform after you have mastered them on the floor.

The exercise planner, found at the back of the book, includes a core stability routine as part of the weekly program, so you can put into action, and benefit from, the exercises included in this chapter.

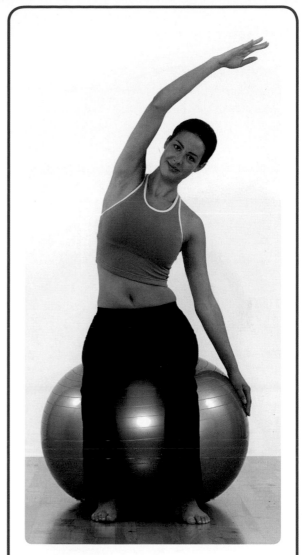

Equipment

The amount of equipment you need is up to you—there are plenty of pieces of equipment that create an unstable base and make your core muscles work really hard. For the purpose of this chapter, we recommend using an exercise ball for variation, but if you don't want to buy one, there are plenty of exercises to choose from to begin with. An exercise mat is also recommended, and small cushions or folded towels make ideal padding during exercises that involve lying on the floor or kneeling.

warming-up exercises

It is always essential to warm up before undertaking any form of exercise. Choose a couple of the exercises shown over the next few pages and spend a little time warming up. You should allow around ten minutes for this, and alternate them so you don't get bored.

standing abdominal hollowing

For all the core stability exercises, you have to activate the deep inner-unit muscles in a hollowing action, so this exercise is an essential part of your warm-up.

1 Stand tall with your feet hips' width apart and your spine in neutral.

2 Pull your stomach muscles in and up to hollow your abdomen, keeping your attention focused on your navel. Imagine that there is a belt around your waist and that you are simply tightening the belt one notch. Hold for a count of five.

3 Perform three repetitions.

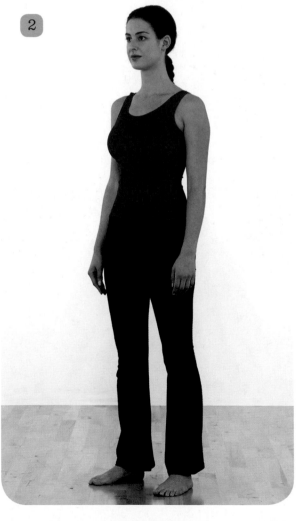

> **PAY ATTENTION**
>
> The action should feel light and subtle—do not hold your breath or suck in your waist because you won't be using your deep stabilizing muscles. Keep your hips, legs and spine still and restrict movement to your stomach muscles alone—try not to flatten your back.

torso rotations

Gradually increase the range of movement as you do this exercise, reaching across your torso with your opposite hand as you do so. The twisting action should force you to come up onto the toes of your opposite foot.

1 Keep your pelvis in neutral and stand with your feet hips' width apart and knees slightly bent.

2 Rotate your torso to one side then the other, increasing the range of movement as you do so. You should feel a slight stretch across your back and shoulders.

3 Perform five to ten turning press repetitions.

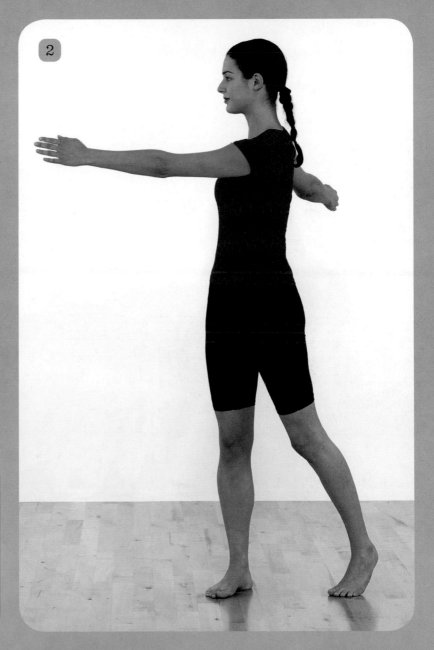

PAY ATTENTION

Always work slowly and with control, and do not push your body farther than it naturally goes—you should not feel any pain or discomfort when doing these exercises. Over time, you will become more flexible and will naturally be able to stretch farther.

full body reach-up

This opens and strengthens your shoulders, lengthens your spine and neck, and improves your posture. Keep your arms straight throughout the exercise.

1 Stand with your feet close together, knees soft, spine in neutral, and abdominal muscles set.

2 Slowly raise your arms up from each side, bringing your palms together above your head.

3 Take your arms back down to the starting position.

4 Repeat the movement five times.

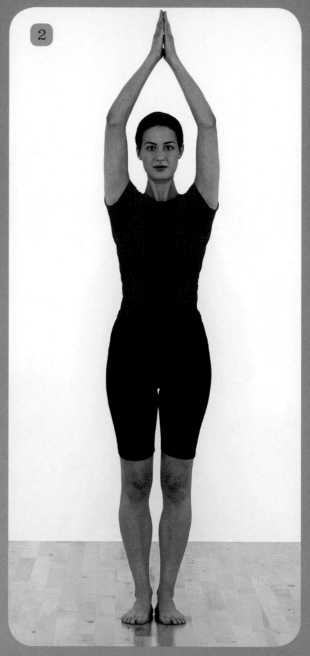

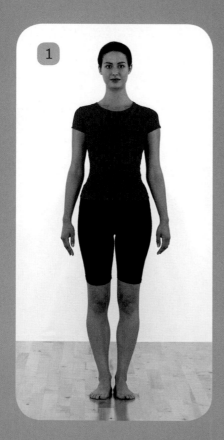

sitting spinal twist

Aim to keep your spine straight without rounding your back.

1 Sit up straight with your legs extended in front of you, knees slightly bent, and feet flexed. Raise your arms to the sides at shoulder height and tighten your abdominal muscles to support your back.

2 Turn your head and shoulders toward your left, keeping your back, hips, and buttocks motionless as you move.

3 Rotate as far as is comfortable, then hold for a count of one. Return to the starting position and repeat on the other side.

4 Repeat on each side, rotating a little farther the easier it becomes.

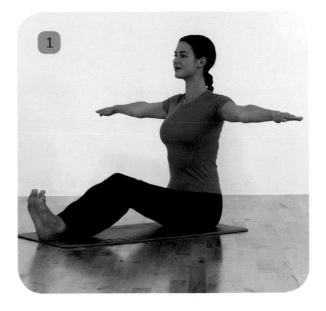

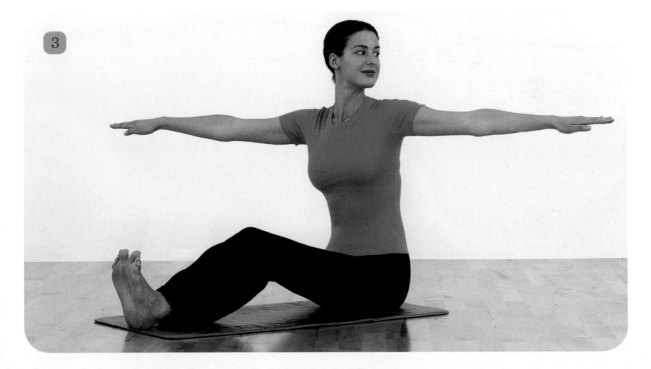

introductory exercises

These first-stage exercises are aimed at beginners, so you should find them relatively easy to start with, allowing you to become more involved as you progress. If you find any of the exercises a bit too difficult, feel free to replace them with something else of the same level.

sitting stomach workout

This tones and flattens your deep stomach muscle (transversus abdominis) and the one that runs down the front of your stomach (the rectus abdominis).

1 Sit forward on a chair. Keep your feet flat on the floor, hips' width apart, with your knees over your ankles and your palms on your thighs.

2 Sit up straight. Tighten the abdominal muscles by gently pulling your navel in toward your spine. Hold for ten seconds, then relax.

3 Rest for a count of three before doing any repetitions.

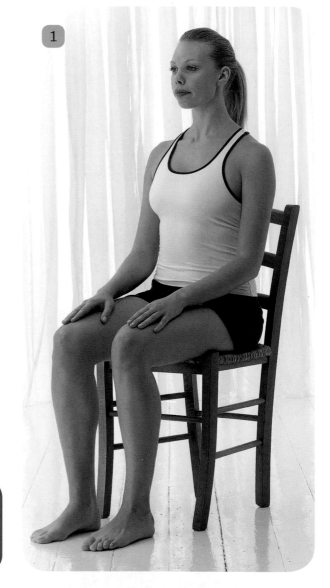

> ## PAY ATTENTION
> Breathe regularly as you do this exercise—don't hold your breath because it will make your blood pressure rise, which can be dangerous when exercising.

squat with leg lift

This move works your entire lower body. Focus on keeping your abdominal muscles braced to maintain your balance.

1 Stand on the floor with your feet parallel and hips' width apart. Place your hands on your hips, set your abdominal muscles, and bend your knees so that you squat back.

2 Press up into a standing position as you simultaneously extend your right leg to the side.

3 Return to the squatting position.

4 Repeat on the other side.

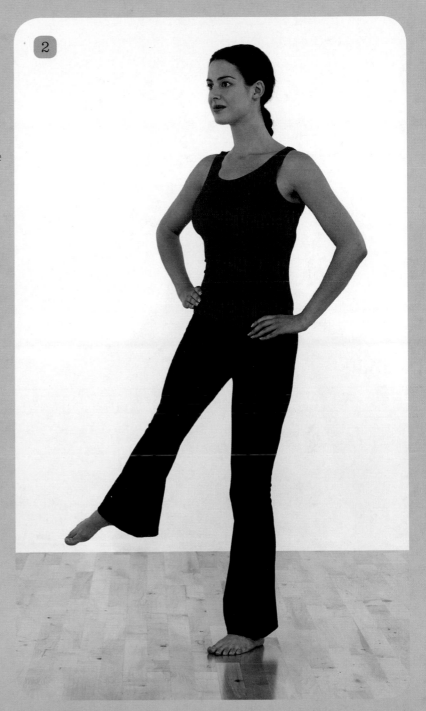

2

stability bridge

You need to perfect this exercise in order to improve the stability of the trunk muscles before you can move on to more challenging movements.

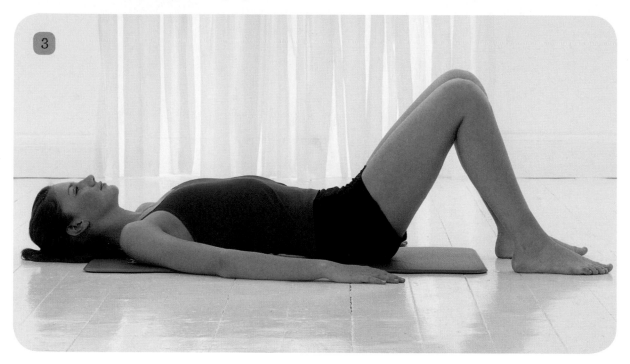

1 Lie on your back with your knees bent and your feet flat on the floor, slightly apart. Keep your arms by your sides, palms facing downward.

2 Tighten your abdominal muscles by gently drawing in your navel toward your spine (which will support your back).

3 Press your lower back down into the floor and gently tilt your pelvis forward so that the pubic bone rises.

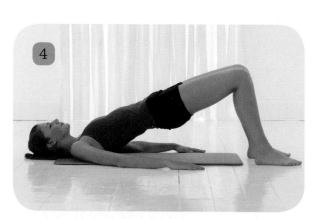

4 Use your hip, thigh, and trunk muscles to lift your pelvis until your body forms a straight line from your shoulders to your knees. Hold for a count of five, then return to the starting position.

oblique press

This is an isometric exercise in which you push against your knee in order to tone the abdominals. It involves a slight turn, so it helps the muscles at the sides of the trunk.

1 Lie on your back, knees bent and feet flat on the floor. Place your arms by your sides. Press your lower back into the floor.

3 Do the same with the other leg and hand, again holding the position for a count of ten.

PAY ATTENTION
Keep your back flat on the floor as you do this exercise.

2 Raise your right leg from the floor so that your thigh is at a 90-degree angle to the floor and your calf is parallel to it. Place the palm of your left hand on your right knee and push against it, resisting the force with your knee so that neither arm nor leg moves position. Hold the position for a count of ten, then relax.

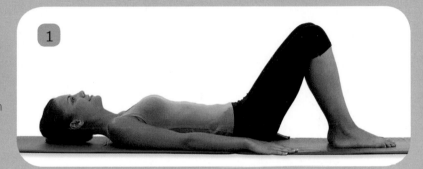

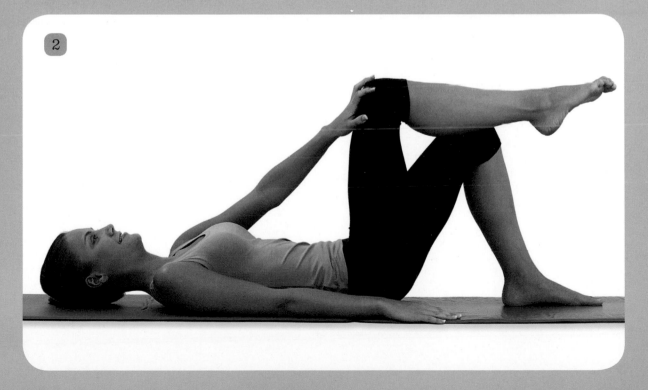

sitting reverse abdominal curl

This is an easy exercise that can be done almost anywhere. It works your rectus abdominis. Try to avoid sagging or arching the back and hold your abdominal muscles in tight throughout the movement.

1 Sit on a stool or on a bench with good posture. Set your abdominal muscles and extend your arms in front of you at shoulder height.

2 Slowly lean your torso and shoulders backward, keeping the spine rigid, as far back as is comfortable.

3 Hold the position for a count of two, then return to the starting position.

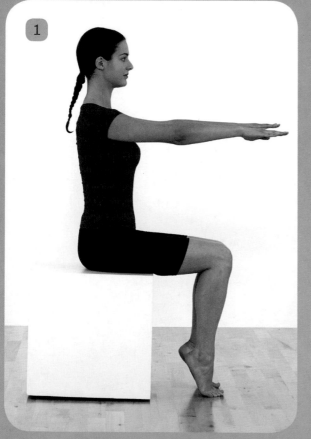

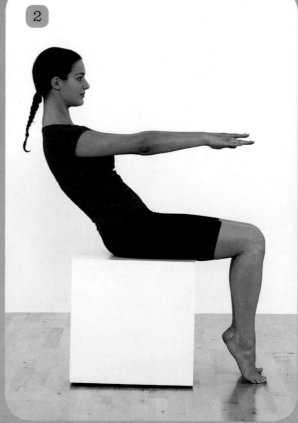

waist twist

Make sure you have a lot of space around you so that when you swing your arms you don't hit anything. This is a fun exercise to do and it really gets to work on the obliques (the muscles at the side of your waist) to help define a curvy silhouette.

1 Stand with feet hips' width apart, hands by sides, and knees slightly bent.

2 Extend your arms out in front of you and form loose fists with both hands.

3 Swing your arms from side to side, making sure your feet stay firmly on the floor and your hips face forward. Start off slowly and then build up speed, making sure you keep control of the movement and your hips stay facing the front.

4 When about 30 seconds are up, drop your arms back down by your sides and return to the starting position.

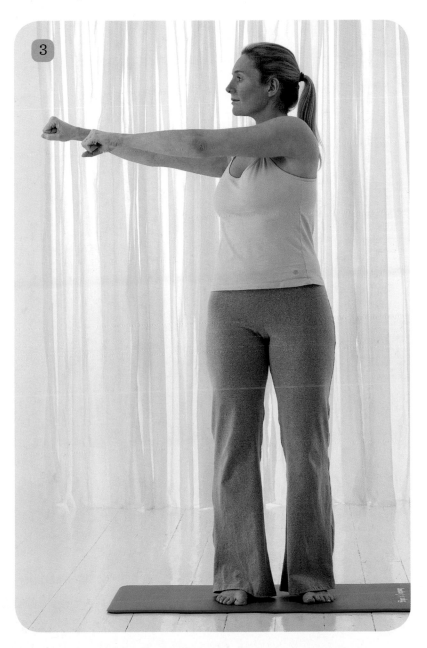

PAY ATTENTION
Don't get carried away while swinging your arms because you may end up pulling a muscle. If you have to go slowly to control the movement, so be it.

mermaid

This exercise works your obliques and increases lateral flexion. Try to keep your spine straight and do not lean forward or backward. If you don't have an exercise ball, you can kneel with your feet under your buttocks instead.

1 Sit up on the ball with good posture, your spine in neutral, and your feet parallel on the floor and hips' width apart. Tighten your abdominal muscles and let your arms rest by your sides.

2 Reach your right arm up to the ceiling and lean over to the left side so that you reach the right arm over your head. Hold for a count of one, then lower your arm.

3 Repeat on the other side.

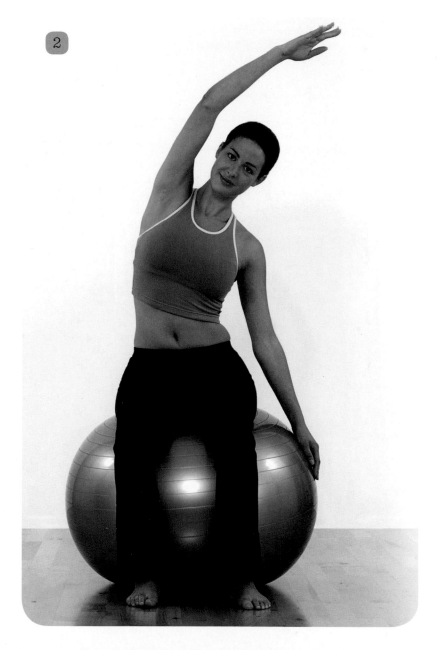

190

single leg stretch

This exercise will help you learn to stabilize your abdominals and hips, and will work your entire abdominal area. It will also stretch your back and legs.

1 Lie on your back with your pelvis in neutral. Bend your knees and rest your feet on an exercise ball. Keep your arms by your sides and rest your head on a flat pillow.

2 Set your abs and raise your right leg into the air up to the ceiling, pressing your left leg into the ball.

3 Bring your right leg down and repeat on the left leg.

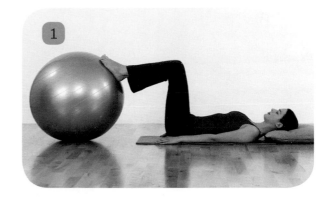

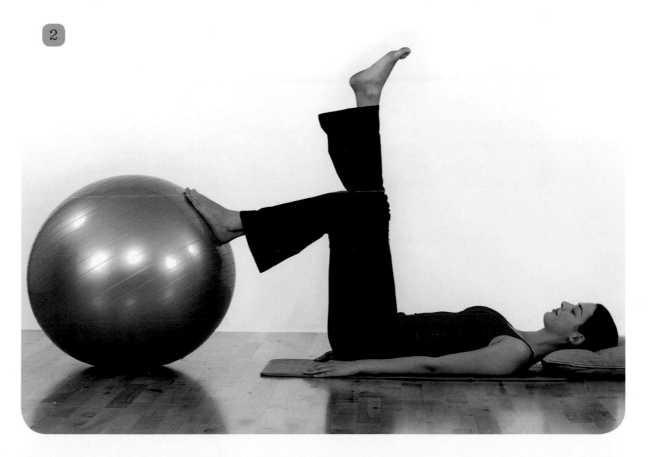

side leg lift

This exercise strengthens your obliques, hips, buttocks, and thighs.

1 Lie on your right side with your legs extended but knees soft, not locked, toes pointed, and your right arm supported by a cushion or pillow. Rest your left hand on the floor in front of you and support the side of your head with your right hand.

2 Keep your spine in neutral and set your abdominal muscles.

3 Turn your left leg out slightly, then raise it toward the ceiling as far as is comfortable. Hold briefly, then slowly release.

4 Repeat on the other side.

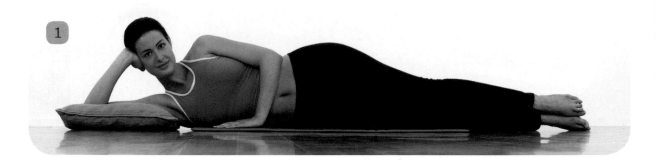

1

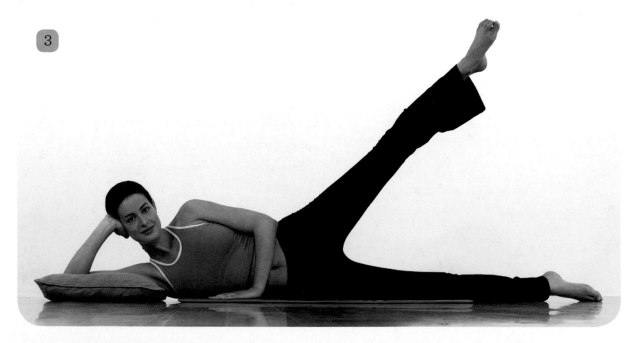

3

side standing leg lift

This works your abdominal muscles and back extensors as well as your quadriceps, hamstrings, and gluteals (buttock muscles).

1 Stand up straight with your spine in neutral, your feet hips' width apart, and arms by your sides. Set your abdominal muscles.

2 Support your body weight on your right leg and lift your left leg to the side. As you do this, extend your right arm forward and your left arm out to the side. Hold for a count of three.

3 Repeat on the other side.

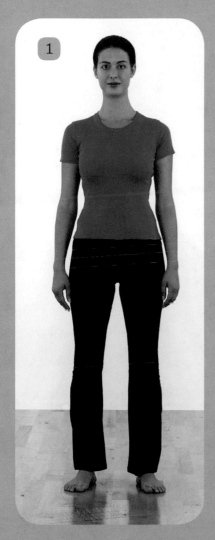

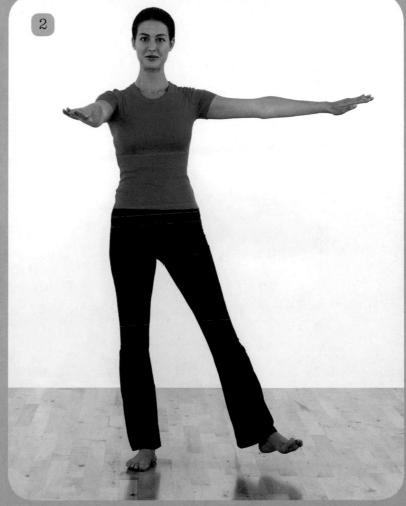

advanced exercises

Now that you've worked through the introductory exercises and are feeling more confident and fitter, you can progress to this second series of exercises. As before, if you find any particular exercises too difficult, feel free to replace them with something else from this level.

dog

This classic yoga position strengthens and stretches most of your body. As your flexibility increases, you will be able to press your heels into the floor.

1 Start on all fours with your hands under your shoulders and your knees under your hips, hip-distance apart. Keep your spine in neutral and slowly tighten your abdominal muscles.

2 Curl your toes under, press back into your palms, and, bringing the balls of your feet onto the floor, lift your hips toward the ceiling and straighten your legs until you are forming an inverted "V" shape.

3 Hold briefly, then come down again on all fours.

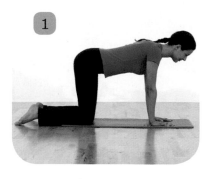

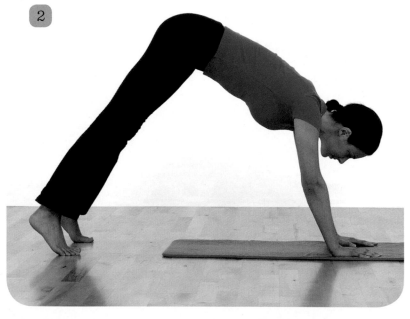

side leg circles

This exercise tones and strengthens your core muscles as well as the hips, buttocks, and inner thighs.

1 Lie on your right side with your head supported by your right hand and your right arm supported by a cushion or pillow. Rest your left hand on the floor in front of you.

2 Bend your right leg in front of you for support.

3 Keep your spine in neutral and set your abdominal muscles.

4 Point your left foot and raise your left leg, raising it as high as feels comfortable. Then draw five small clockwise circles with your toes, keeping your abs strong throughout and moving from your hip joint.

5 Reverse the direction and draw five small anticlockwise circles, then slowly release.

6 Repeat on the other side.

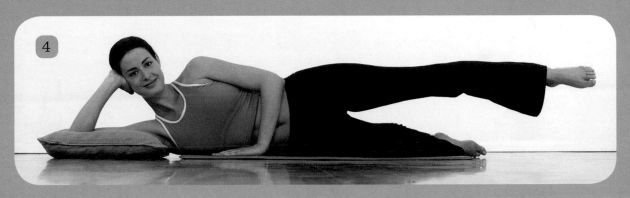

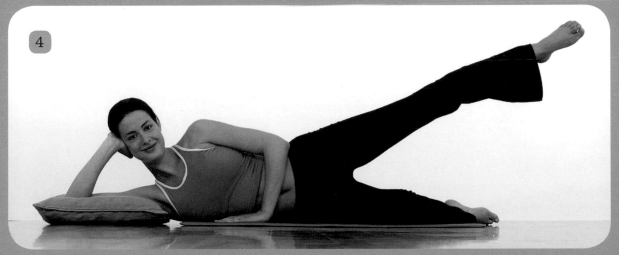

reverse bridge on an exercise ball

This exercise improves your balance while working your abdominal muscles, lower back, pelvic stabilizers, gluteals, and hamstring muscles.

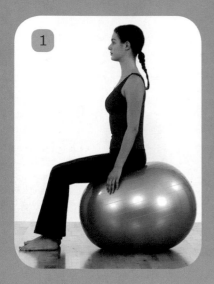

1 Sit on the ball with your hands by your sides and feet on the floor, hips' width apart.

2 Walk your feet forward, rolling your hips down and lying back on the ball as you do so. Stop when your shoulder blades are on the ball.

3 Lower your head to the ball and lift your hips so that your torso is in a straight line, tightening your abdominal muscles as you do so. Hold for a count of ten.

4 Slowly drop your hips and lift your head off the ball.

5 Walk your feet back, pressing your lower back into the ball as you go, and return to the start position to finish.

PAY ATTENTION

To increase the difficulty of this exercise, you can raise and lower alternate legs once you are in position.

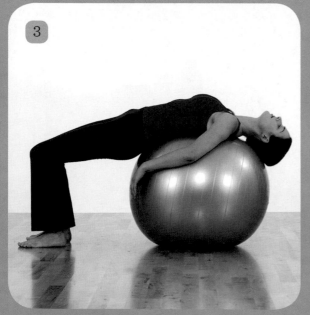

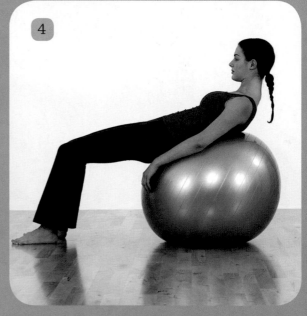

ball rotation

This exercise should only be attempted when you can perform reverse bridges on an exercise ball with confidence. Just do the exercise once to start with, and then add repetitions when you can do it easily.

1 Roll into position as if you were doing a reverse bridge. Lie with the ball beneath your shoulders, keep your spine in neutral, and tighten your abdominal muscles.

2 Hold your arms out to the sides. Slowly walk sideways so that the ball moves from one shoulder to the other, then repeat to the other side.

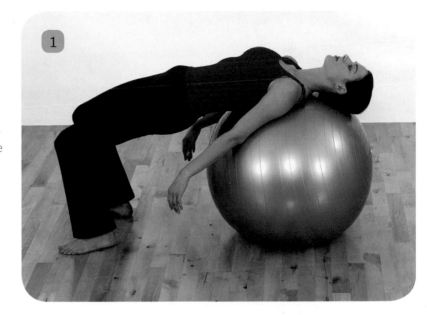

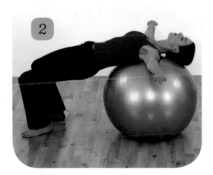

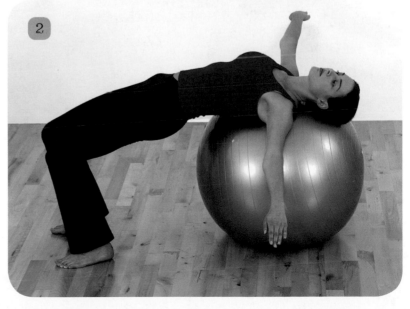

standing leg lift

This will help improve your balance, stabilize the pelvis, and tone your thigh and hip muscles. Aim to keep your pelvis stable throughout.

1 Stand with your spine in neutral, feet slightly apart and arms by your sides.

2 Pull your navel in toward your spine and bring your left knee in toward your chest so that your big toe is resting on the side of your right knee. Hold your knee with both hands, keeping your spine straight and your standing leg strong. You will need to drop your left hip down and lift the hip higher on the right side to keep your hips level at this point.

3 Hold for a count of three, then release. Repeat with the other leg.

4 To make this exercise more difficult, after step 2 stretch your left leg straight out in front of you at hip height, holding onto the back of your thigh to support it. Release your arms and rest them on your buttocks, but keep your left leg extended in front of you. Hold for up to ten seconds, then lower your leg to the floor and repeat on the other leg.

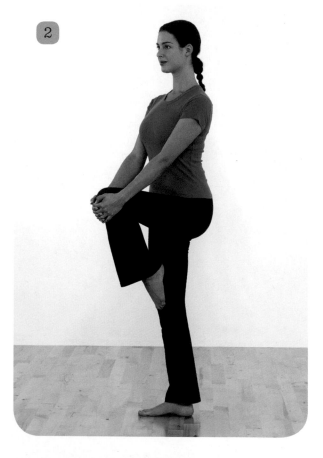

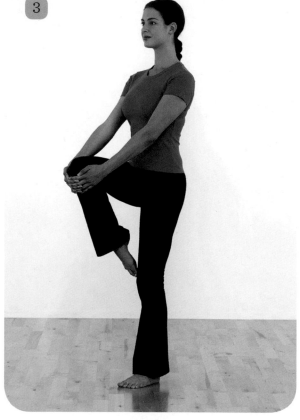

double leg stretch

This exercise will make your deep stabilizing muscles work to control the weight and movement of your legs. Along with strengthening your deep abdominal muscles and inner thigh muscles, this exercise aims to build a strong center, which remains stable when you move your arms and legs.

1 Lie on your back with your knees bent and your arms by your sides.

2 Keep your spine in neutral and tighten your abdominal muscles. Pick up the exercise ball between your ankles and squeeze together, pulling your knees toward you.

3 Gently sit up far enough so that you are resting your upper body on your elbows.

4 Straighten your legs out diagonally and hold for a count of five. Return to the starting position.

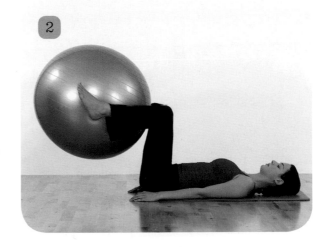

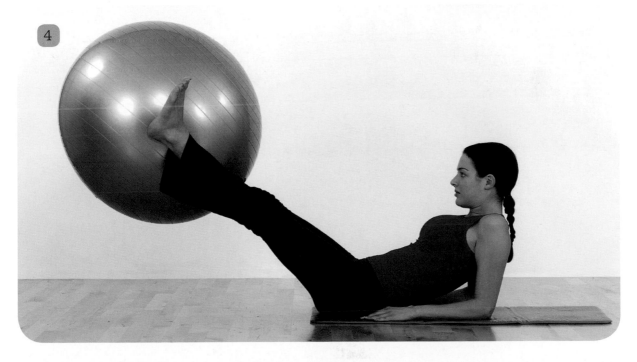

swan

This lengthens and strengthens your spine, as well as works your abs. To maintain the tension in your abdominals during this exercise, imagine that you are trying to lift your stomach off the ground.

1 Lie on your front with your arms extended in front of you and your legs extended behind.

2 Keep your spine in neutral and tighten your abdominal muscles. You should feel your pubic bone pressing down into the floor.

3 Raise your shoulders and feet a few inches off the ground and hold for a count of ten, then release.

2

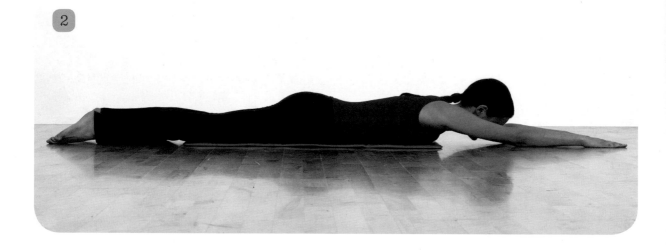

3

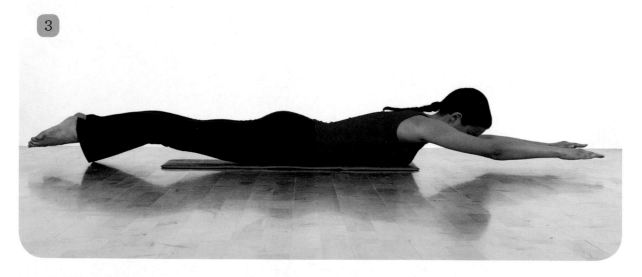

swan variation

Performing this move on an exercise ball strengthens and stretches your back. If you can feel any discomfort in your lower back, stop immediately.

1 Lie with the ball under your stomach and pelvis. Plant your curled toes on the floor, hips' width apart, and keep your legs straight. Place your hands on the floor, shoulders' width apart.

2 Tighten your abdominal muscles and lift your head so that there is a long line from your head to your heels. Slowly push your pelvis into the ball as you look up and extend your spine away from the ball. Hold for a count of five, then release.

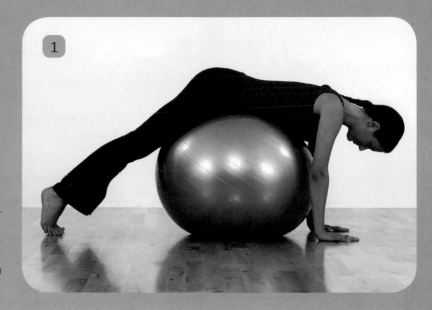

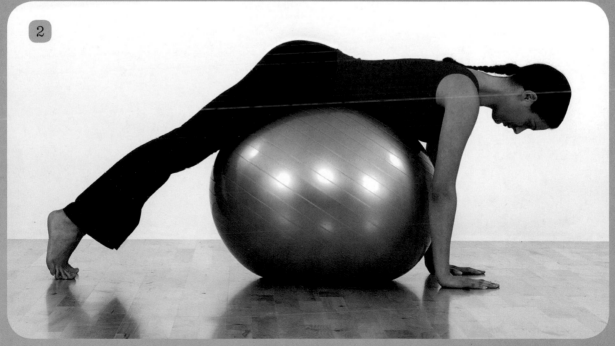

supine leg lift

The importance of this exercise is to hold the legs off the floor with correct spinal alignment and abdominal bracing. You can use small ankle weights for extra challenge.

1 Lie on your back with your knees bent and feet on the floor, hip-distance apart.

2 Keep your spine and pelvis in neutral and gently tighten your abdominal muscles.

3 Keeping your knees bent, slowly lift your right leg several inches off the floor and hold it.

4 Now bring your left leg off the floor and bring it adjacent to the right leg.

5 Slowly lower your right leg back to the floor, then the left leg.

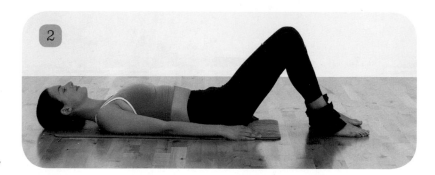

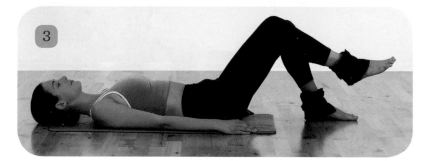

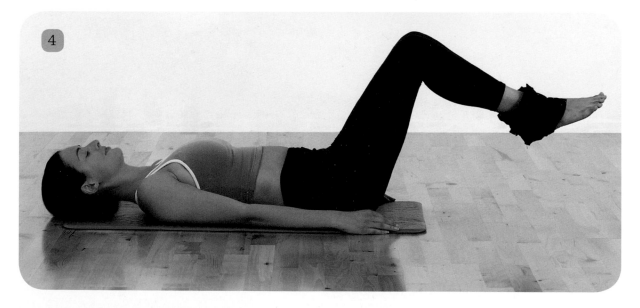

rolling like a ball

This exercise improves your balance and the flexibility of your spine and builds strong abdominal muscles.

1 Sit up with your knees bent and hold your knees with your hands. Pull your abdominal muscles toward your spine to help keep your balance. Tuck your chin into your chest and, staying balanced on your tailbone, lift both feet off the floor.

2 Roll back slowly, bringing your knees closer to your nose, until your shoulder blades touch the floor, making sure you do not roll back onto your neck. Then roll forward to the starting position.

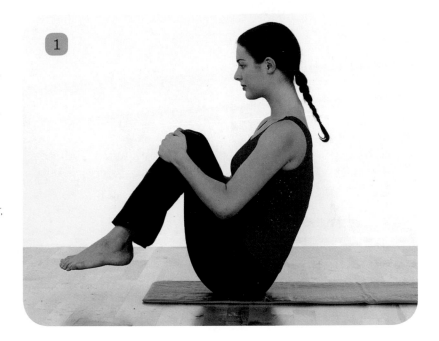

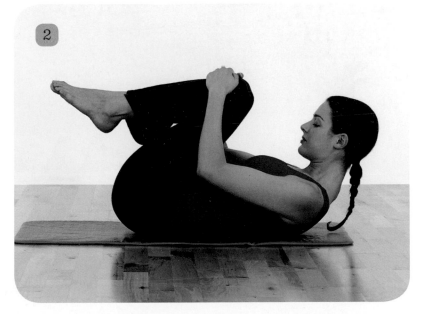

PAY ATTENTION

Focus on moving from your abdominal muscles instead of letting momentum carry you backward.

cooling-down exercises

Just as you need to warm up the body for exercising, you also need to cool it down after you have finished. Choose a few of the exercises shown over the next six pages, and take the time to cool down. Ideally, you should look to spend around ten minutes doing this.

swimming stretch

This exercise mimics the movements used during walking. It's good preparation for keeping the lower back still when you are walking in daily life.

1 Lie on your back, knees bent, feet flat on the floor, and your arms by your sides. Arch your back and then flatten it. Find the midway neutral position between the two extremes.

2 Lift your right arm and extend it backward. At the same time, extend your left leg. Hold the position for a count of five, then return your arm and leg to the starting position. Repeat up to ten times.

3 Now do the same on the other side, extending your left arm and your right leg. Again hold the position for a count of five, then return to the starting position.

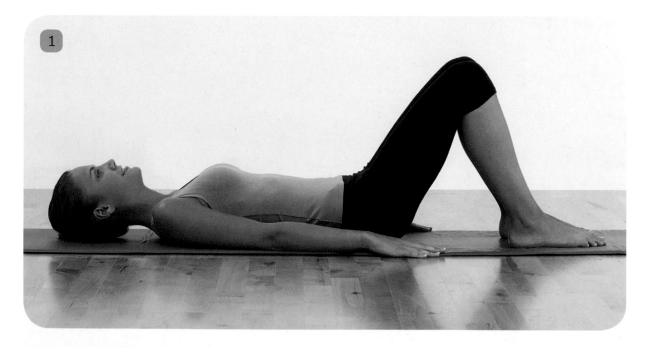

sitting spinal stretch

This movement stretches and rotates your abdomen, ribs, and spine and stretches your hip muscles. Make sure you move from your hips up, not from your shoulders down.

1 Sit up straight with your legs out in front of you. Bend your right knee and pull your right foot into your left buttock.

2 Bend your left knee and place your left foot on your right knee.

3 Gently draw your navel in toward your spine to set your abdominal muscles and slowly rotate to the left. Use your left hand to help keep your body upright. Rotate as far as is comfortable and hold the stretch for at least a count of 15.

4 Release and return to the start position, then rearrange your legs so that your right one is on top and rotate to the other side of your body.

> **PAY ATTENTION**
> Aim to keep your spine straight throughout this move and don't arch your back.

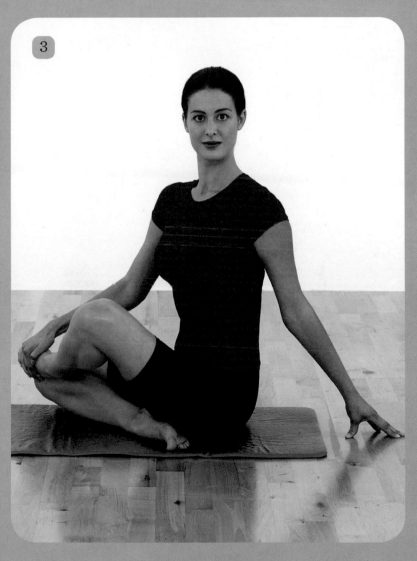

oblique stretch

This is an easy way to give the muscles in your waist a really good stretch. As you walk your hands around to get into position, you may not be able to reach your knees but that's fine—just go as far around as you can comfortably.

1 Get down on the floor on all fours with your knees resting directly below your hips and your hands below your shoulders.

2 Keeping your knees where they are, walk both your hands around to your right-hand side to meet your knees, so you are twisting from the waist. You should feel the stretch down your left-hand side. Hold the stretch for ten seconds, then walk the hands back around to the starting position.

3 Repeat the movement so you are stretching around to the left-hand side.

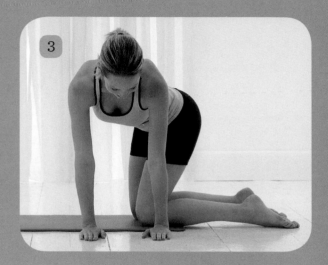

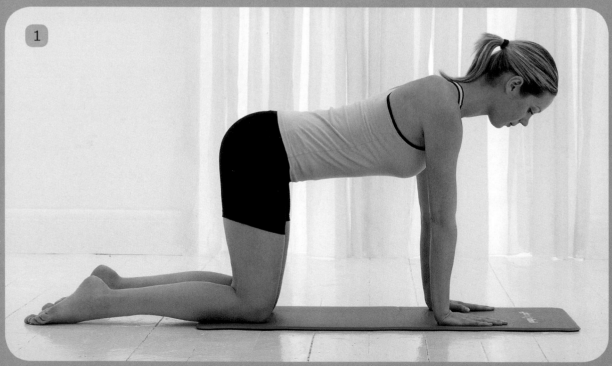

knee hug

This will stretch and release the muscles in your lower back.

1 Lie on your back with your legs in the air and your knees bent. Tighten your abdominal muscles to protect your lower back.

2 Lift your knees to your chest and hold onto your shins.

3 Pull your knees in as tightly as is comfortable and hold for at least 15 seconds. Slowly release, return to the start position, and repeat.

> **Quality control**
> Focus on perfecting your technique—it's the quality of the movements that will count. Remember to keep your spine aligned and your abdominal muscles pulled in at all times.

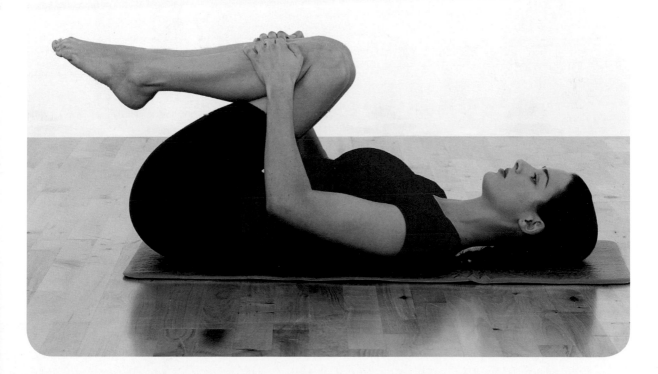

cat stretch

This stretch is known as the cat stretch because you look a lot like a cat if you do it right! It targets most of the major muscles in the back.

1 Get down on the floor on all fours. Let your head and neck relax so they are in line with your spine and you are looking down toward the floor.

2 Slowly arch your back by pulling in your stomach muscles and pushing the curve of your spine toward the ceiling. Tilt your head and neck up toward the ceiling as you do this.

3 Hold the stretch for around eight seconds, then lower your back so it's straight and in the starting position again. While you do this, let your head and neck relax.

4 Pause for a brief moment, then repeat three times.

5 When you have finished, lean back onto your heels and stretch your arms out in front of you—this completes the movement.

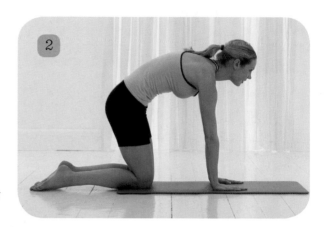

> **PAY ATTENTION**
> Try not to let your back sag because this could cause serious back injuries. You can avoid this by doing the stretch slowly and gently to make sure you are in control at all times.

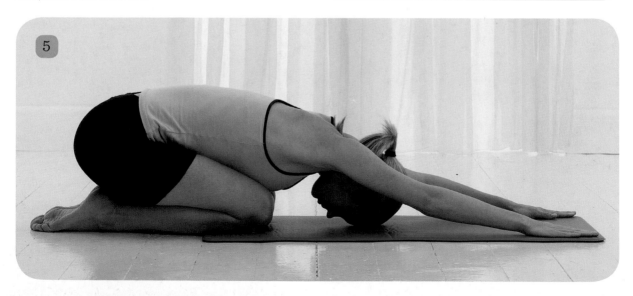

side stretch

This is great for stretching the upper body, but stretch only as far is comfortable.

1 Kneel on your left knee and straighten your right leg out to the side.

2 Put your left hand on the floor and bring your right arm over your head until you feel a stretch in your side. Do not overstretch.

3 Hold for a count of ten, then return to the starting position. Repeat on the other side of the body.

Top tips for superstretching

- Only stretch warm muscles.
- Slowly ease the muscle into position.
- Do not bounce into position.
- Never overstretch—mild discomfort is acceptable but if it hurts, you should stop.
- Don't hold your breath—breathing freely will enable blood to flow to the muscles.

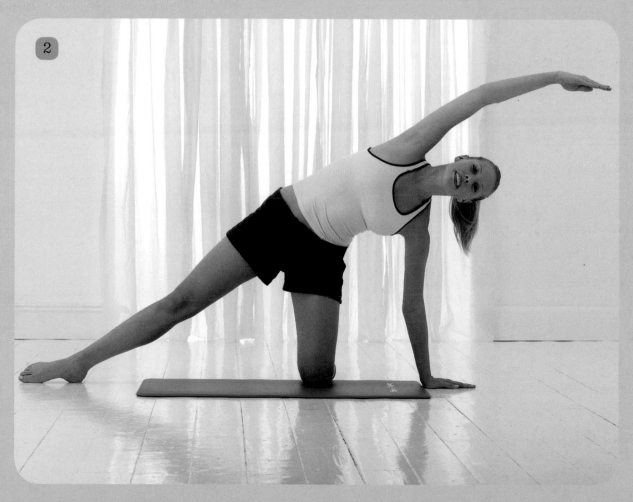

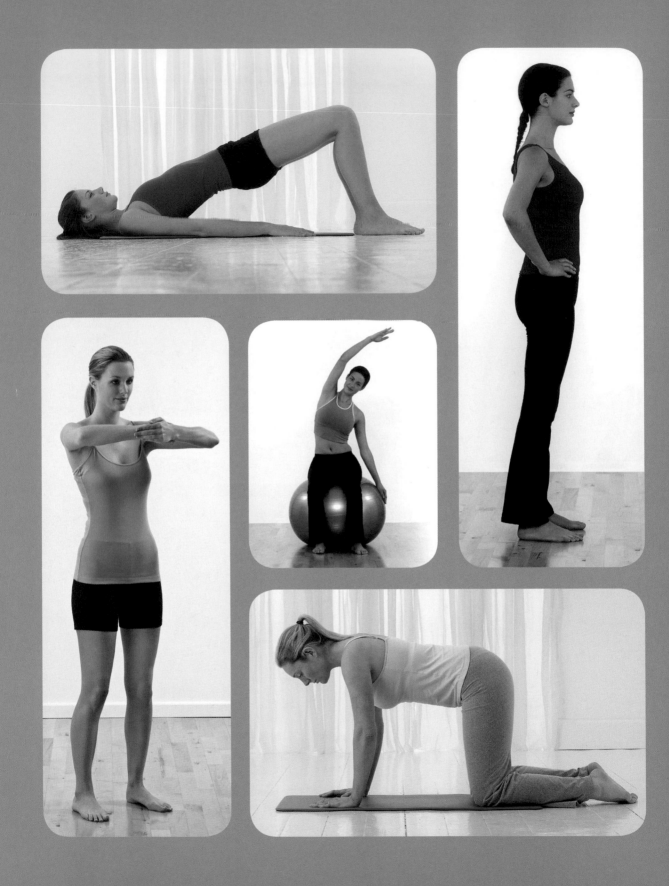

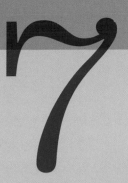

exercise planner

Here's where it all comes together, the 12-week planner. Although the sessions are broken down into daily routines for you to follow, if you're new to exercise, don't feel you have to start off doing the whole routine—you can build up the amount of time you spend and the types of exercises you do. So no more excuses about starting tomorrow or next week—there's no time like today!

introductory exercises

Here is your starter six-week plan. We recommend that you begin with and follow the introductory exercises before embarking on the advanced sessions. Make sure that each day you warm up before the exercise routine, and at the end allow time to cool down and stretch.

To start, aim to do one or two sets of eight repetitions for each exercise. Don't feel you have to complete the whole routine—you can build up the amount of reps as you progress.

week 1
one or two sets of eight reps

DAY 1 chest & back
easy plank p. 42
c-curve p. 43
standing wall push-up p. 44
back arch p. 45
bust lift p. 46
bell pull p. 47

DAY 2 arms & shoulders
sitting back toner p. 76
biceps curl p. 77
triceps squeeze back p. 78
turning press p. 79
front raises p. 79
front arm toner (hammer curl) p. 80

DAY 3 stomach
belly tightener p. 112
side reach p. 113
sitting knee lift p. 114
spine rotation p. 115
reverse curl p. 116
basic oblique curl p. 117

DAY 4 legs & buttocks
basic squat p. 148
buttock walking p. 149
standing calf raises p. 150
stepping p. 151
bridge squeeze p. 152
kneeling kickback p. 153

DAY 5 core stability
sitting stomach workout p. 184
squat with leg lift p. 185
stability bridge p. 186
oblique press p. 187
sitting reverse abdominal curl p. 188
waist twist p. 189

DAY 6 legs & buttocks
buttock walking p. 149
superman p. 154
inner thigh lift p. 155
outer thigh lift p. 156
kneeling kickback p. 153
straight leg outer thigh lift p. 157

DAY 7 mixed combination
easy plank p. 42
standing wall push-up p. 44
biceps curl p. 77
triceps extension p. 82
basic squat p. 148
sitting reverse abdominal curl p. 188

Keeping up your motivation

When you start your program, be realistic about how and when you can do it. You do need to set aside a regular slot for your routine so it becomes a natural and automatic part of your everyday life, just like brushing your teeth. But if you do miss several days, don't get disheartened and give up—a little exercise even on a very irregular basis is still better than nothing at all!

week 2
one or two sets of eight reps

DAY 1 stomach
belly tightener p. 112
side reach p. 113
sitting knee lift p. 114
spine rotation p. 115
reverse curl p. 116
basic oblique curl p. 117

DAY 2 chest & back
back arch p. 45
bust lift p. 46
crisscross arms p. 48
prayer p. 49
easy chest flex p. 50
boxing p. 51

DAY 3 legs & buttocks
bridge squeeze p. 152
kneeling kickback p. 153
superman p. 154
inner thigh lift p. 155
outer thigh lift p. 156
straight leg outer thigh lift p. 157

DAY 4 stomach
spine rotation p. 115
reverse curl p. 116
leg slide p. 118
simple pelvic tilt p. 119
abdominal curl p. 120
moving curl p. 121

DAY 5 arms & shoulders
biceps curl p. 77
triceps squeeze back p. 78
superwoman arms p. 81
triceps extension p. 82
kneeling box push-up p. 83
side shoulder raise p. 84

DAY 6 core stability
stability bridge p. 186
oblique press p. 187
mermaid p. 190
single leg stretch p. 191
side leg lift p. 192
side standing leg lift p. 193

DAY 7 mixed combination
boxing p. 51
kneeling box push-up p. 83
abdominal curl p. 120
basic squat p. 148
bridge squeeze p. 152
side standing leg lift p. 193

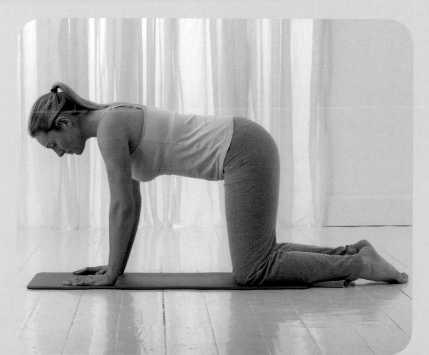

Reps—weeks 1–3
One repetition equals one exercise, following the step-by-step instructions. A set is a group of repetitions and at this point of the program we advise that you complete one to two sets of eight repetitions for each exercise.

week 3
one or two sets of eight reps

DAY 1 **legs & buttocks**

basic squat p. 148

buttock walking p. 149

stepping p. 151

kneeling kickback p. 153

inner thigh lift p. 155

outer thigh lift p. 156

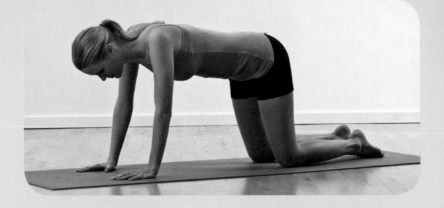

DAY 2 **chest & back**

easy plank p. 42

standing wall push-up p. 44

bust lift p. 46

bell pull p. 47

crisscross arms p. 48

boxing p. 51

DAY 3 **arms & shoulders**

biceps curl p. 77

turning press p. 79

front arm toner (hammer curl) p. 80

superwoman arms p. 81

kneeling box push-up p. 83

triceps ponytail p. 85

DAY 5 **stomach**

belly tightener p. 112

side reach p. 113

reverse curl p. 116

basic oblique curl p. 117

abdominal curl p. 120

moving curl p. 121

DAY 4 **core stability**

squat with leg lift p. 185

stability bridge p. 186

oblique press p. 187

waist twist p. 189

single leg stretch p. 191

side leg lift p. 192

DAY 6 **chest & back**

c-curve p. 43

back arch p. 45

bust lift p. 46

crisscross arms p. 48

prayer p. 49

easy chest flex p. 50

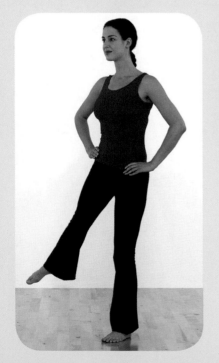

Don't rest too much

Don't stop for more than a minute between exercises. Shorter recovery periods result in better muscles all around and improved muscle endurance. Keep it up!

DAY 7 **mixed combination**

easy plank p. 42

biceps curl p. 77

belly tightener p. 112

straight leg outer thigh lift p. 157

sitting reverse abdominal curl p. 188

side standing leg lift p. 193

making progress

Well done, you have reached the point of the first six-week program where you should now be feeling fitter and are becoming familiar with the various exercises. Time to step up the work rate a little, so each session is now three to four sets of eight repetitions.

Don't forget, make sure that each day you warm up before the exercise routine, and at the end allow time to cool down and stretch.

week 4
three or four sets of eight reps

DAY 1 **chest & back**
easy plank p. 42
c-curve p. 43
standing wall push-up p. 44
back arch p. 45
bust lift p. 46
bell pull p. 47

DAY 2 **arms & shoulders**
sitting back toner p. 76
biceps curl p. 77
triceps squeeze back p. 78
turning press p. 79
front raises p. 79
front arm toner (hammer curl) p. 80

DAY 3 **stomach**
belly tightener p. 112
side reach p. 113
sitting knee lift p. 114
spine rotation p. 115
reverse curl p. 116
basic oblique curl p. 117

DAY 4 **legs & buttocks**
basic squat p. 148
buttock walking p. 149
standing calf raises p. 150
stepping p. 151
bridge squeeze p. 152
kneeling kickback p. 153

DAY 5 **core stability**
sitting stomach workout p. 184
squat with leg lift p. 185
stability bridge p. 186
oblique press p. 187
sitting reverse abdominal curl p. 188
waist twist p. 189

DAY 6 **legs & buttocks**
buttock walking p. 149
standing calf raises p. 150
superman p. 154
inner thigh lift p. 155
outer thigh lift p. 156
straight leg outer thigh lift p. 157

DAY 7 **mixed combination**
easy plank p. 42
standing wall push-up p. 44
biceps curl p. 77
triceps extension p. 82
basic squat p. 148
sitting reverse abdominal curl p. 188

Working your muscles

The aim of these programs is to make your muscles work harder, either by increasing the time you exercise or by increasing the intensity of your workout. Your muscles will start to become tired during the last repetitions and you may feel a burning sensation in the area you're working on, but this is normal and will pass as soon as you rest.

week 5
three or four sets of eight reps

DAY 1 stomach
belly tightener p. 112
side reach p. 113
sitting knee lift p. 114
spine rotation p. 115
reverse curl p. 116
basic oblique curl p. 117

DAY 2 chest & back
back arch p. 45
bust lift p. 46
crisscross arms p. 48
prayer p. 49
easy chest flex p. 50
boxing p. 51

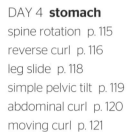
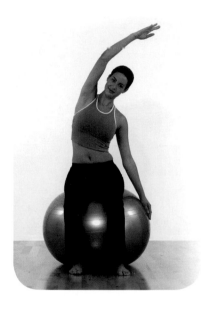

DAY 3 legs & buttocks
bridge squeeze p. 152
kneeling kickback p. 153
superman p. 154
inner thigh lift p. 155
outer thigh lift p. 156
straight leg outer thigh lift p. 157

Reps—weeks 4-6
Now you are progressing well we
advise that you complete three to
four sets of eight repetitions for
each exercise.

DAY 4 stomach
spine rotation p. 115
reverse curl p. 116
leg slide p. 118
simple pelvic tilt p. 119
abdominal curl p. 120
moving curl p. 121

DAY 5 arms & shoulders
biceps curl p. 77
triceps squeeze back p. 78
superwoman arms p. 81
triceps extension p. 82
kneeling box push-up p. 83
side shoulder raise p. 84

DAY 6 core stability
stability bridge p. 186
oblique press p. 187
mermaid p. 190
single leg stretch p. 191
side leg lift p. 192
side standing leg lift p. 193

DAY 7 mixed combination
boxing p. 51
kneeling box push-up p. 83
abdominal curl p. 120
basic squat p. 148
bridge squeeze p. 152
side standing leg lift p. 193

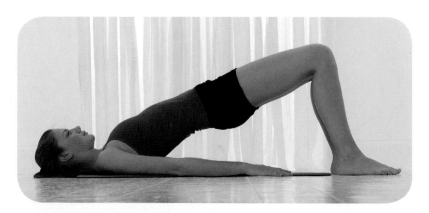

week 6
three or four sets of eight reps

DAY 1 legs & buttocks
basic squat p. 148
buttock walking p. 149
standing calf raises p. 150
stepping p. 151
inner thigh lift p. 155
outer thigh lift p. 156

DAY 2 chest & back
easy plank p. 42
standing wall push-up p. 44
bust lift p. 46
bell pull p. 47
crisscross arms p. 48
boxing p. 51

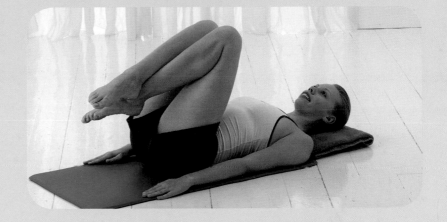

DAY 3 arms & shoulders
biceps curl p. 77
turning press p. 79
front arm toner (hammer curl) p. 80
superwoman arms p. 81
kneeling box push-up p. 83
triceps ponytail p. 85

DAY 4 core stability
squat with leg lift p. 185
stability bridge p. 186
oblique press p. 187
waist twist p. 189
single leg stretch p. 191
side leg lift p. 192

DAY 5 stomach
belly tightener p. 112
side reach p. 113
reverse curl p. 116
basic oblique curl p. 117
abdominal curl p. 120
moving curl p. 121

DAY 6 chest & back
c-curve p. 43
back arch p. 45
bust lift p. 46
crisscross arms p. 48
prayer p. 49
easy chest flex p. 50

DAY 7 mixed combination
easy plank p. 42
biceps curl p. 77
belly tightener p. 112
straight leg outer thigh lift p. 157
sitting reverse abdominal curl p. 188
side standing leg lift p. 193

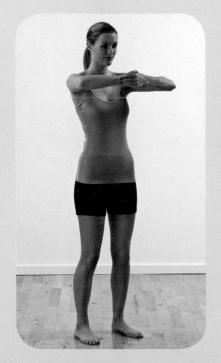

Setting the pace
It's important to work at the right intensity—put in too little effort and you won't notice much difference; throw yourself into the exercises and you may hurt yourself.

advanced exercises

Now you have worked through the introductory exercises, you are ready to embark on the advanced sessions. Make sure that each day you warm up before the exercise routine, and at the end allow time to cool down and stretch.

Begin with one or two sets of eight repetitions for each exercise. By now you will know what you are capable of, so work at your own pace and build up the level of repetitions as you progress.

week 7
one or two sets of eight reps

DAY 1 chest & back
plank p. 52
super chest toner p. 53
open flyer p. 54
front-lying chest lift p. 55
moy complex p. 56
bent-over arm shaper p. 57

DAY 2 arms & shoulders
arms out biceps curl p. 86
triceps kickback p. 87
box push-up (advanced) p. 88
standing long arm palm press p. 89
circles in the air p. 90
triceps bend p. 91

DAY 3 stomach
crunches p. 122
side lift p. 123
bicycle p. 124
lower abdominal raise p. 125
slightly harder reverse curl p. 126
pillow roll p. 127

DAY 4 legs & buttocks
wide squat p. 158
lunge p. 159
double knee bends p. 160
front leg raise p. 161
scissors p. 162
one leg knee bends p. 163

DAY 5 core stability
dog p. 194
side leg circles p. 195
ball rotation p. 197
standing leg lift p. 198
double leg stretch p. 199
swan p. 200

DAY 6 stomach
crunches p. 122
side lift p. 123
toe touch p. 128
"hundreds" p. 129
slightly harder oblique curl p. 130
leg lift p. 131

DAY 7 mixed combination
open flyer p. 54
moy complex p. 56
box push-up (advanced) p. 88
triceps bend p. 91
front leg raise p. 161
double leg stretch p. 199

Taking it farther
Don't forget, if you want to get fit, then you'll have to include some activity that raises your heartbeat for at least 15 minutes at a time. Swimming, cycling, fast walking, and running are all straightforward options, but you could do an exercise class or take up a sport, such as tennis, if you like—just keep moving and try a variety of activities.

week 8
one or two sets of eight reps

DAY 1 legs & buttocks
double knee bends p. 160
front leg raise p. 161
leg lift p. 164
straight leg inner thigh lift p. 165
one leg buttock clencher p. 166
bridge with leg lift p. 167

DAY 2 arms & shoulders
triceps kickback p. 87
box push-up (advanced) p. 88
arm opener p. 92
upright pull p. 93
triceps dips p. 94
floor arm lift p. 95

DAY 3 chest & back
super chest toner p. 53
front-lying chest lift p. 55
dumbbell row p. 58
chest press p. 59
reverse sit-up p. 60
soup-can press p. 61

DAY 4 stomach
bicycle p. 124
lower abdominal raise p. 125
toe touch p. 128
"hundreds" p. 129
slightly harder oblique curl p. 130
leg lift p. 131

DAY 5 core stability
reverse bridge on an exercise ball
   p. 196
standing leg lift p. 198
double leg stretch p. 199
swan variation p. 201
supine leg lift p. 202
rolling like a ball p. 203

DAY 6 legs & buttocks
wide squat p. 158
lunge p. 159
double knee bends p. 160
front leg raise p. 161
scissors p. 162
one leg knee bends p. 163

DAY 7 mixed combination
dumbbell row p. 58
triceps dips p. 94
crunches p. 122
toe touch p. 128
double knee bends p. 160
bridge with leg lift p. 167

Reps—weeks 7–9
These exercises are a little more difficult; for the first three weeks you should complete one to two sets of eight repetitions for each exercise.

How to breathe properly
Breathe in slowly through your nose, and notice how the top of the abdomen rises as you do so. Hold the breath for a few seconds, then breathe out slowly through your mouth.

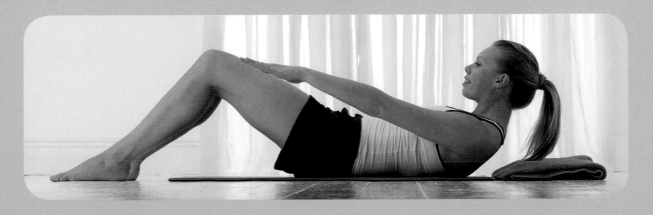

week 9
one or two sets of eight reps

DAY 1 stomach

crunches p. 122

side lift p. 123

lower abdominal raise p. 125

slightly harder reverse curl p. 126

toe touch p. 128

"hundreds" p. 129

DAY 2 chest & back

super chest toner p. 53

front-lying chest lift p. 55

moy complex p. 56

bent-over arm shaper p. 57

dumbbell row p. 58

chest press p. 59

DAY 3 arms & shoulders

triceps kickback p. 87

standing long arm palm press p. 89

circles in the air p. 90

triceps bend p. 91

triceps dips p. 94

floor arm lift p. 95

DAY 4 core stability

side leg circles p. 195

standing leg lift p. 198

double leg stretch p. 199

swan p. 200

supine leg lift p. 202

rolling like a ball p. 203

DAY 5 legs & buttocks

wide squat p. 158

lunge p. 159

double knee bends p. 160

front leg raise p. 161

leg lift p. 164

bridge with leg lift p. 167

DAY 6 chest & back

plank p. 52

open flyer p. 54

moy complex p. 56

chest press p. 59

reverse sit-up p. 60

soup-can press p. 61

DAY 7 mixed combination

arms out biceps curl p. 86

box push-up (advanced) p. 88

slightly harder oblique curl p. 130

straight leg inner thigh lift p. 165

one leg buttock clencher p. 166

dog p. 194

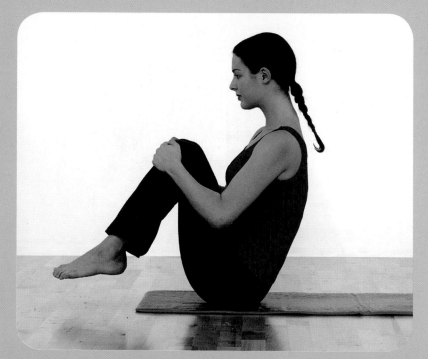

Keep going!

Building muscle tone doesn't happen overnight, but the beauty of these short routines is that you won't become bored or burned out. Keep it up and you'll find that just a short routine once a day really will make a difference.

really making progress!

Fantastic, you have reached the halfway point of the second six-week program. You should now be feeling pretty fit, and the exercises are part of your daily life. At this point you are ready to increase the work rate, so each session is now three to four sets of eight repetitions.

As always, make sure that each day you warm up before the exercise routine, and at the end allow time to cool down and stretch.

week 10
three or four sets of eight reps

DAY 1 **chest & back**
plank p. 52
super chest toner p. 53
open flyer p. 54
front-lying chest lift p. 55
moy complex p. 56
bent-over arm shaper p. 57

DAY 2 **arms & shoulders**
arms out biceps curl p. 86
triceps kickback p. 87
box push-up (advanced) p. 88
standing long arm palm press p. 89
circles in the air p. 90
triceps bend p. 91

DAY 3 **stomach**
crunches p. 122
side lift p. 123
bicycle p. 124
lower abdominal raise p. 125
slightly harder reverse curl p. 126
pillow roll p. 127

DAY 4 **legs & buttocks**
wide squat p. 158
lunge p. 159
double knee bends p. 160
front leg raise p. 161
scissors p. 162
one leg knee bends p. 163

DAY 5 **core stability**
dog p. 194
side leg circles p. 195
ball rotation p. 197
standing leg lift p. 198
double leg stretch p. 199
swan p. 200

DAY 6 **stomach**
crunches p. 122
side lift p. 123
toe touch p. 128
"hundreds" p. 129
slightly harder oblique curl p. 130
leg lift p. 131

DAY 7 **mixed combination**
open flyer p. 54
moy complex p. 56
box push-up (advanced) p. 88
triceps bend p. 91
front leg raise p. 161
double leg stretch p. 199

Stomach muscles
Apart from the obvious benefit of improving your appearance, firming and toning up your stomach muscles is actually good for you. It will improve your posture and balance and increase your flexibility, helping to keep your body in good working order as you get older.

week 11
three or four sets of eight reps

DAY 1 **legs & buttocks**
double knee bends p. 160
front leg raise p. 161
leg lift p. 164
straight leg inner thigh lift p. 165
one leg buttock clencher p. 166
bridge with leg lift p. 167

DAY 2 **arms & shoulders**
triceps kickback p. 87
box push-up (advanced) p. 88
arm opener p. 92
upright pull p. 93
triceps dips p. 94
floor arm lift p. 95

DAY 3 **chest & back**
super chest toner p. 53
front-lying chest lift p. 55
dumbbell row p. 58
chest press p. 59
reverse sit-up p. 60
soup-can press p. 61

DAY 4 **stomach**
bicycle p. 124
lower abdominal raise p. 125
toe touch p. 128
"hundreds" p. 129
slightly harder oblique curl p. 130
leg lift p. 131

DAY 5 **core stability**
reverse bridge on an exercise ball
  p. 196
standing leg lift p. 198
double leg stretch p. 199
swan variation p. 201
supine leg lift p. 202
rolling like a ball p. 203

DAY 6 **legs & buttocks**
wide squat p. 158
lunge p. 159
double knee bends p. 160
front leg raise p. 161
scissors p. 162
one leg knee bends p. 163

DAY 7 **mixed combination**
dumbbell row p. 58
triceps dips p. 94
crunches p. 122
toe touch p. 128
double knee bends p. 160
bridge with leg lift p. 167

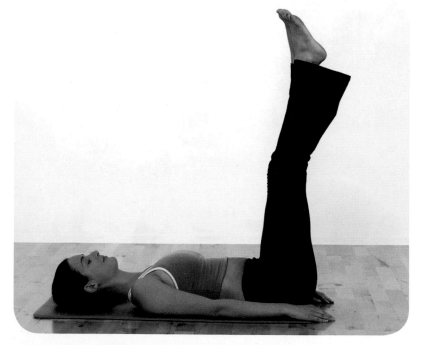

Repetitions

Muscle-building exercises are done
as a series of repetitions. To build
strength and endurance, you need
to repeat the same exercise again
and again. The aim is to work until
your muscles feel tired, and over
time this will strengthen them so
that they can work harder.

week 12
three or four sets of eight reps

DAY 1 stomach
crunches p. 122
side lift p. 123
lower abdominal raise p. 125
slightly harder reverse curl p. 126
toe touch p. 128
"hundreds" p. 129

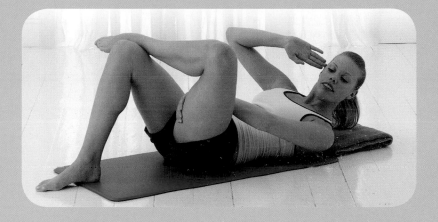

DAY 2 chest & back
super chest toner p. 53
front-lying chest lift p. 55
moy complex p. 56
bent-over arm shaper p. 57
dumbbell row p. 58
chest press p. 59

DAY 3 arms & shoulders
triceps kickback p. 87
standing long arm palm press p. 89
circles in the air p. 90
triceps bend p. 91
triceps dips p. 94
floor arm lift p. 95

DAY 6 chest & back
plank p. 52
open flyer p. 54
moy complex p. 56
chest press p. 59
reverse sit-up p. 60
soup-can press p. 61

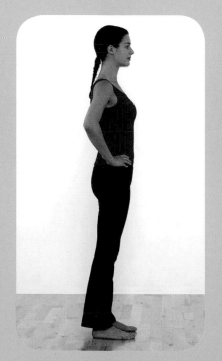

DAY 4 core stability
side leg circles p. 195
standing leg lift p. 198
double leg stretch p. 199
swan p. 200
supine leg lift p. 202
rolling like a ball p. 203

DAY 7 mixed combination
arms out biceps curl p. 86
box push-up (advanced) p. 88
slightly harder oblique curl p. 130
straight leg inner thigh lift p. 165
one leg buttock clencher p. 166
dog p. 194

DAY 5 legs & buttocks
wide squat p. 158
lunge p. 159
double knee bends p. 160
front leg raise p. 161
leg lift p. 164
bridge with leg lift p. 167

Reps—weeks 10-12
Now you are really feeling the benefits, you should be able to step up to three to four sets of eight repetitions for each exercise.

maintaining the program

If during the plan you find yourself having one of those "Why bother?" days, sit down and spend time finding an inspiring thought to lift your spirits.

Remind yourself why you are doing the exercises. Maybe it's because you want to wear a cropped top again on your vacation, perhaps you want to feel more confident in how you look, or you want to get rid of the surplus bulge around your midriff that is so reluctant to move.

Taking on an exercise plan is not meant to be an ordeal. Yes, you will have to be prepared for a little hard work at times, but it should not be something you dread doing. It is important that you persevere with the program—so here are some thoughts and ideas for keeping on track, and also, making you feel good about yourself.

Don't give up!

Exercise is easy to let slip when you're feeling under the weather, and it's fine to give your body a break every now and then. But, if you ever feel like you want to give up, read these top motivational tips:

• Visualize how you will look and feel if you stick to the program instead of letting it slip. It should be enough to spur you on.

• Remember that a few minutes for exercise will not encroach greatly on your time. You'll feel much more alert for doing the workout, and it will pay dividends in the long run.

• Not only is exercising good for your body but it's good for your mind, too. So, even if you're feeling down, it's the perfect thing to do!

Thinking positive

You may well face days during your program when you are plagued by negative thoughts, but hidden beneath those dull feelings are positive emotions lying in wait. So work hard each day to bring them to the fore. When you feel good about yourself, you can begin to understand and accept the type of person you are and not punish yourself mentally for any shortcomings or imperfections. We are all human, after all. Experts have found that people who are positive and optimistic enjoy long-term good health.

Inspiring words

When working through your program, keep these six motivational sentences in mind each time you feel your willpower sagging:

I will keep focused, and by the end I will:
• feel healthier
• feel more confident
• feel better about how I look in snug-fitting clothes
• want to wear short cropped tops
• not have a bad back
• enjoy improved posture

By the end of the program, with perseverance and dedication, you will have achieved every one of them.